Management of the
High Risk Infant
Beyond Survival

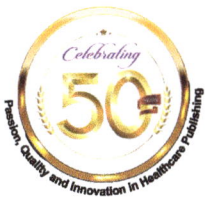

Management of the
High Risk Infant
Beyond Survival

Sudha Chaudhari
Consultant
Department of Pediatrics
Terre Des Hommes Rehabilitation and
Morris Child Development Centre
King Edward Memorial Hospital
Pune, Maharashtra, India

Foreword
Haresh Kirpalani

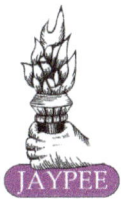

JAYPEE BROTHERS MEDICAL PUBLISHERS
The Health Sciences Publisher
New Delhi | London

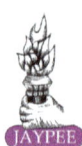 **Jaypee Brothers Medical Publishers (P) Ltd.**

Headquarters
Jaypee Brothers Medical Publishers (P) Ltd
EMCA House, 23/23-B
Ansari Road, Daryaganj
New Delhi 110 002, India
Landline: +91-11-23272143, +91-11-23272703
+91-11-23282021, +91-11-23245672
E-mail: jaypee@jaypeebrothers.com

Corporate Office
Jaypee Brothers Medical Publishers (P) Ltd
4838/24, Ansari Road, Daryaganj
New Delhi 110 002, India
Phone: +91-11-43574357
Fax: +91-11-43574314
E-mail: jaypee@jaypeebrothers.com

Overseas Office
JP Medical Ltd
83 Victoria Street, London
SW1H 0HW (UK)
Phone: +44 20 3170 8910
Fax: +44 (0)20 3008 6180
E-mail: info@jpmedpub.com

Website: www.jaypeebrothers.com
Website: www.jaypeedigital.com

© 2021, Jaypee Brothers Medical Publishers

The views and opinions expressed in this book are solely those of the original contributor(s)/author(s) and do not necessarily represent those of editor(s) of the book.

All rights reserved. No part of this publication may be reproduced, stored or transmitted in any form or by any means, electronic, mechanical, photocopying, recording or otherwise, without the prior permission in writing of the publishers.

All brand names and product names used in this book are trade names, service marks, trademarks or registered trademarks of their respective owners. The publisher is not associated with any product or vendor mentioned in this book.

Medical knowledge and practice change constantly. This book is designed to provide accurate, authoritative information about the subject matter in question. However, readers are advised to check the most current information available on procedures included and check information from the manufacturer of each product to be administered, to verify the recommended dose, formula, method and duration of administration, adverse effects and contraindications. It is the responsibility of the practitioner to take all appropriate safety precautions. Neither the publisher nor the author(s)/editor(s) assume any liability for any injury and/or damage to persons or property arising from or related to use of material in this book.

This book is sold on the understanding that the publisher is not engaged in providing professional medical services. If such advice or services are required, the services of a competent medical professional should be sought.

Every effort has been made where necessary to contact holders of copyright to obtain permission to reproduce copyright material. If any have been inadvertently overlooked, the publisher will be pleased to make the necessary arrangements at the first opportunity. The **CD/DVD-ROM** (if any) provided in the sealed envelope with this book is complimentary and free of cost. **Not meant for sale.**

Inquiries for bulk sales may be solicited at: jaypee@jaypeebrothers.com

Management of the High Risk Infant: Beyond Survival

First Edition: **2021**

ISBN: 978-93-90020-72-0

Dedicated to

My husband Dr Vijay Chaudhari
for his unwavering support in all my endeavors

Contributors

Aditi Patwardhan
Associate Consultant
Department of Ophthalmology
King Edward Memorial Hospital
Pune, Maharashtra, India

Ashima Choudhari
Fellow in Pediatric Orthopedics
King Edward Memorial Hospital
Pune, Maharashtra, India

Bharati Patil
Head
Department of Occupational Therapy
Terre Des Hommes Rehabilitation and
Morris Child Development Centre
King Edward Memorial Hospital
Pune, Maharashtra, India

Bindu Patni
Head
Child Development Centre
Terre Des Hommes Rehabilitation and
Morris Child Development Centre
King Edward Memorial Hospital
Pune, Maharashtra, India

Neelam Vaid
Associate Professor and
Consultant (ENT)
King Edward Memorial Hospital
Pune, Maharashtra, India

Rakesh Meena
Fellow in Pediatric Orthopedics
King Edward Memorial Hospital
Pune, Maharashtra, India

Sameer Desai
Associate Consultant
Department of Pediatric Orthopedics
King Edward Memorial Hospital
Pune, Maharashtra, India

Shweta Deshpande
Assistant Professor (Audiology)
School of Audiology and Speech
Language Pathology (SASLP)
Bharatiya Vidyapeeth
(Deemed to be University)
Pune, Maharashtra, India

Sudha Chaudhari
Consultant
Department of Pediatrics
Terre Des Hommes Rehabilitation and
Morris Child Development Centre
King Edward Memorial Hospital
Pune, Maharashtra, India

Foreword

It is my distinct pleasure to provide this foreword. This book on follow-up of vulnerable newborns in the Indian context is extremely important in my view. It comes from an eminent neonatal follow-up physician—one who has pioneered the implementation of follow-up practices in India. High attrition rate of follow-up is a major source of bias for all outcome statistics. The challenges of overcoming this to minimize bias are self-evidently higher in India than elsewhere. Dr Sudha Chaudhari has shown how attrition rates can in practice be lowered in India.

Why is this important? There are at least three reasons why this is very relevant to practice within India.

First, the explosion of high technology medicine now extends most sharply into intensive care medicine. Naturally, newborn intensive care has benefitted from the dramatic new possibilities. But all such advances are fraught with potential for harm as well as good. Perhaps it is a classic case of a double-edged sword. These advances cannot be simply implemented with purely a "technical gaze." They must be evaluated. But how are they to be so evaluated? In today's perinatology, we have come a long way in understanding that short-term gain—let us say survival at all costs—is not necessarily adequate. Increasingly, we as a worldwide community understand that the gain is to be expressed as a metric summarizing both survival and quality of survival. This could be addressed in posing the question, "With what sequelae is that survival achieved?" It then becomes immediately obvious that this requires follow-up of the newborn infant. But this is easier said than done. How are relevant follow-up programs to be instituted in the India of today? Such questions are considered in this book.

Second, and following directly from the first—is the enormous sociological dimension of the follow-up outcomes of vulnerable preterm infants. In any society, this is a huge question, and one that is often tacitly ignored. But is it one that can be wisely ignored anywhere? In Western countries, there has been an implicit—I doubt it can be said to be explicit—general agreement that all advances be made widely and as soon as they can be practically disseminated. In the aftermath of the COVID-19 pandemic, even the richest countries are likely to have to grapple more explicitly with this. If that is true in the richest countries, what about in India? But of course one cannot resolve such discussion without knowing the specifics in any particular country. That means, knowing what the follow-up is in India, and facilitating programs for follow-up.

This leads directly to the third issue—that of India specific long-term follow-up. Of what relevance is the outcome of 22 weekers' gestation in Japan or Sweden—in counseling a parent in any part of India? The particular outcomes of complex processes of care may primarily reflect the disease process and other purely universal biological variables. But obviously they also depend upon specifics of the particular population, and the particular hospital or care setting. This has three corollaries. The first is that it is not adequate to simply stake off the shelf studies from very differing societal and care structures, to apply outcome statistics to India. Second, for parents in India, long-term prognosis and relevant counseling has to be based on local data. Finally, if quality improvement is to continue making the strides it has in India, it needs longer term outcomes.

Dr Sudha has intimate knowledge of these dimensions. She has been continuously funded by the Indian Council of Medical Research since 1987 up to 2012. She continues to be involved in cutting-edge research to this day—with her collaborators in the "Pune Low Birth Weight Study". Moreover, she has trained scores of young professionals on the importance and techniques of good follow-up practice. Having confronted the practical as well as theoretical issues involved, she is in a unique position to advise the future of follow-up of Indian preterms. Finally, I must make a personal observation that arises from when she and I first met. She spotted me looking anxiously in the entrance of King Edward Memorial Hospital, Pune, Maharashtra, India, as jet-lagged as I was, searching for my sick father. She demonstrated so much compassion and guided me around. Undoubtedly, she has the compassion needed to underpin the necessary science. Either one (science or compassion) alone, one without the other is at the end of the day, simply many words. The two together make for a better future.

Haresh Kirpalani MD MSc
Emeritus Professor (Pediatrics)
McMaster University
Ontario, Canada
Emeritus Professor
The Children's Hospital of Philadelphia University of Pennsylvania
Philadelphia, Pennsylvania, USA

Preface

I joined King Edward Memorial Hospital, Pune, as a Consultant 45 years ago. At that time, our neonatal unit was situated in one corner of the Obstetric Ward. We had six "so-called" incubators, which were essentially plastic boxes. We had light bulbs on pulleys, so if the baby got cold, we pulled the bulb down, if the baby got hot we pulled the bulb up.

In 1981, we moved to a separate 24-bed neonatal unit, which was the largest neonatal unit in Pune at that time. We started saving smaller and smaller babies. At this point, I realized that there was absolutely no Indian data on what happens to these infants later on in life. Fortunately for us, we had started the Terre Des Hommes Rehabilitation Centre, Morris Child Development Centre, 2 years ago. Another heartening occurrence was that Dr Pramila Phatak, who had published the Indian version of Bayley scales, joined us after retiring from Vadodara.

At a time when pediatricians were busy thinking about malnutrition, Indian childhood cirrhosis, and infectious diseases, Dr Anand Pandit conceived this idea of a center for the "special child," with the principle that every facility for diagnosis and treatment should be available under one roof. The mural at the entrance of the TDH Center symbolized our philosophy. About Dr Pandit, I would say, "excellence can be achieved if you risk more than what others think is safe, and dream more than what others think is practical." This book would not have been possible without the facilities of this center.

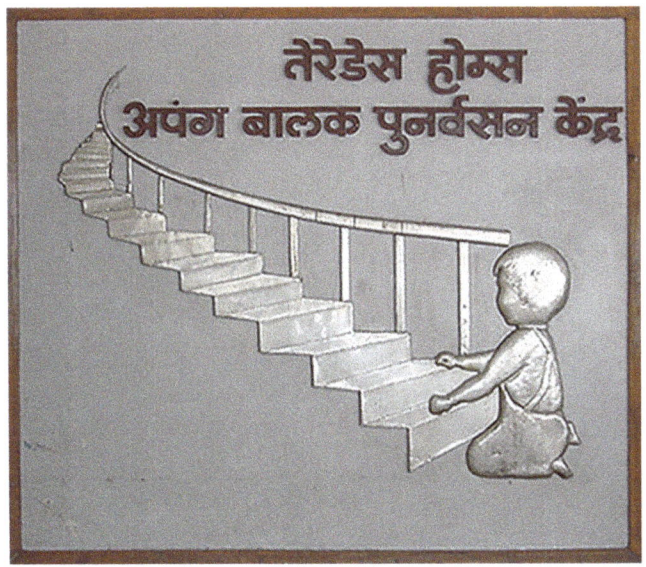

We encourage this "special child" to climb these stairs and achieve his/her maximum potential.

In 1987, we applied for a grant to Indian Council of Medical Research (ICMR), New Delhi, for the research project, "Pune Low Birth Weight Study: Birth to Adulthood." Although this study is from the preventilation era and the statistics is not relevant today, the methodology is worth emulating for the young neonatologists. It also gives an insight into all the tests that are available in India. This study was supposed to end at 18 years. After reading Professor Barker's studies, I realized that the "Metabolic Syndrome" was seen in 30–40 years old adults who were born small for gestational age (SGA). About 60% of my cohort was SGA and we all know that India is experiencing a burgeoning epidemic of type II diabetes. So the study was extended to 22 years, to look for early predictors of the metabolic syndrome.

We have been doing a 6-day workshop on "High-risk Follow-up and DASII" for the last 10 years and have trained many neonatologists, pediatricians, and psychologists from all over India. Over the years, many participants used to say that there is no Indian book which gives practical aspects of follow-up and Western books on this subject are not relevant to us. So finally, I took the plunge. We have many Sick Newborn Care Units (SNCUs) in smaller towns where pediatric therapists are not available. So the chapter on occupational therapy has explicit instructions with many figures, showing the specific exercises. This book is not a didactic, theoretical book on the subject, but a chronicle of my 40 years' experience in this field. I have tried to make this book a practical guide with many photographs for those who want to start a follow-up program.

I am thankful to Dr Haresh Kripalani for the flattering foreword. I am extremely grateful to our Secretary, Premalatha Raman, who patiently tolerated all my demands, and our computer wizard, Rajesh Jadhav, for all the photographs and technology support. Finally, I am thankful to all the "High-risk Infants" who made this book possible.

This book has been written during the COVID-19 lockdown, which made my life bearable and productive.

Sudha Chaudhari
chaudharisudha2014@gmail.com

Contents

1. **Strategies to Change Neonatal Intensive Care Practices Harmful to the Developing Brain** 1
   Sudha Chaudhari
   - Noise 2
   - Light 2
   - Pain 2
   - Tactile Stimuli 3
   - Medications 3
   - Radiation 4
   - Developmentally Supportive Humanized Care 4

2. **Discharge Planning and Counseling** 6
   Sudha Chaudhari
   - Planning the Discharge 6
   - Discharge Documentation 7
   - Discharge Screening 7
   - Counseling 7
   - Follow-Up 10

3. **Organization of the High-risk Clinic** 13
   Sudha Chaudhari
   - Patient Selection 13
   - Criteria for Close Monitoring 13
   - Functions and Goals of the High-risk Clinic 14
   - Interventions 14
   - Assessments 15
   - Referral to Other Services 16
   - Staff Requirements 16
   - How to Cut Costs? 16
   - Early Intervention 17
   - Schedule of Visits 17
   - Recordkeeping 17
   - Is the Expense Justified? 18

4A. **Hearing Assessment in Infants** 20
   Neelam Vaid, Shweta Deshpande
   - The Hearing Brain 20
   - Causes of Hearing Loss in Infants 21
   - Hearing Assessment 22
   - Screening Techniques 24
   - Diagnostic Tests for Hearing Assessment 26

- Behavioral Assessment *27*
- Electrophysiological Measures *28*
- Exceptional Considerations/Cases *30*

4B. Intervention in Children with Hearing Loss 33
Neelam Vaid, Shweta Deshpande
- Medical/Surgical Intervention *33*
- Types of Hearing Devices *34*
- Aural Habilitation *37*

5A. Visual Impairment 39
Aditi Patwardhan
- Epidemiology: Retinopathy of Prematurity *39*
- Prevalence of Retinopathy of Prematurity in India *39*
- Risk Factors for Retinopathy of Prematurity *40*
- Pathophysiology of Retinopathy of Prematurity *40*
- Classification of Retinopathy of Prematurity *40*
- Disease Location into Zones *41*
- Disease Stages *41*
- Extent of Retinopathy *44*
- Screening for Retinopathy of Prematurity *44*
- Treatment *46*
- Etrop Guidelines for Retinopathy of Prematurity Laser *47*
- Laser Treatment *47*
- Surgical Management of Retinopathy of Prematurity *49*
- Other Causes of Visual Impairment *50*

5B. Retinopathy of Prematurity in a Tertiary Care Center: Incidence, Risk Factors, and Follow-up 52
Sudha Chaudhari

6A. Growth and Development 54
Sudha Chaudhari
- Growth Expectations *54*
- Growth Outcome *54*
- Growth Patterns *54*
- Neurodevelopmental Assessment *56*
- Amiel-Tison Neurological Assessment *57*
- Transient Tone Abnormalities *63*
- Qualitative and Quantitative Assessment *63*
- Precocious Achievement of Motor Milestones *65*
- Developmental Tests *65*
- Investigations *68*

6B. Developmental Assessment Scales for Indian Infants (DASII) 72
Bindu Patni
- Motor Clusters *75*
- Mental Clusters *75*

- Standardization *78*
- Psychometric Properties *78*
- Administration Time *78*
- Administration Procedure *78*
- Scoring *79*

6C. Bayley Scales of Infant and Toddler Development: Third Edition (Bayley III) 81
Bindu Patni
- Cognitive Scale *81*
- Language Scale *82*
- Motor Scale *82*
- Standardization *83*
- Psychometric Properties *83*
- Administration Time *83*
- Scoring *83*

7. Cerebral Palsy 86
Sudha Chaudhari
- Tone *86*
- Children with Athetosis *86*
- Children with Ataxia *86*
- Topographic Classification *87*
- Severity *87*
- Importance of Early Intervention *97*

8A. Early Intervention 99
Sudha Chaudhari

8B. Occupational Therapy with Emphasis on a Home-based Stimulation Program 104
Bharati Patil
- Therapy Plan *106*
- Techniques for Normalizing Tone *106*
- Home-based Stimulation Program *106*
- Development of Hand Function *111*

8C. Orthopedic Management in Cerebral Palsy 115
Sameer Desai, Rakesh Meena, Ashima Choudhari
- Diagnosis and Classification *115*
- Physical Examination of a Child with Cerebral Palsy *116*
- Tone *116*
- Modified Ashworth Scale *117*
- Muscle Strength Analysis and Selective Motor Control *119*
- Concept of Lever Arm Dysfunction and Torsional Profile *119*
- Classification of Cerebral Palsy *120*
- Musculoskeletal Pathology Management *121*
- Botulinum Toxin A *121*
- Orthopedic Surgical Intervention *123*

- Knee Flexion Deformity *124*
- Hip Subluxation and Dislocation *124*
- Scoliosis *125*

9. **Learning Disabilities in Low Birth Weight Children** **128**
   Sudha Chaudhari
   - Incidence *128*
   - Reading Disorder (Dyslexia) *128*
   - Disorder of Written Expression (Dysgraphia) *129*
   - Mathematics Disorder (Dyscalculia) *129*
   - Prediction *132*
   - Importance of Early Diagnosis *133*
   - Red Flag Signs for Learning Disabilities *133*
   - Treatment *134*

10. **Parenting a Child with Disability** **135**
    Sudha Chaudhari

11. **Pune Low Birth Weight Study: Birth to 22 Years** **138**
    Sudha Chaudhari

12. **Pune Neurodevelopmental Screening Test** **153**
    Sudha Chaudhari
    Neurological Examination of Newborns
    and Infants in Office Practice *154*

13. **A Parents' Perspective** **159**
    As narrated by the mother to Dr Sudha Chaudhari

Annexures

Annexure I: Neurological Assessment in the First Year 165

Annexure II: Combined Neurological Assessment of
Neonatologist and Occupational Therapist 170

Annexure III: High-risk Follow-up Clinic:
Neurological Assessment 174

Annexure IV: Stimulation Program for Infants 177

Index *185*

Strategies to Change Neonatal Intensive Care Practices Harmful to the Developing Brain

CHAPTER

Sudha Chaudhari

INTRODUCTION

An increasing number of babies with birth weight <1,000 g [extremely low birth weight (ELBW)] are being saved with the help of drugs such as surfactant and the advances in modern technology. It has been reported that 40% ELBW babies have neurodevelopmental impairment.[1] So, it is extremely important that we devise strategies to decrease the incidence of this impairment by changing some of the practices in the neonatal intensive care unit (NICU) which are harmful to the developing brain.

We do not completely understand the series of events which can cause neurodevelopmental impairment, because it is very complex. It is probably the combination of neonatal care practices and some adverse perinatal events. Gressens et al. demonstrated this "two hit" mechanism in a mouse model.[2] There may be pre-existing lesions in the brain, which may get exacerbated by deleterious factors in the NICU. This will also disrupt normal programming of the brain.

A threefold increase in brain volume, a fourfold increase in cortical gray matter, and a fivefold increase in myelinated white matter occurs between 29 and 40 weeks of gestation. It has been possible to demonstrate this increase with volumetric magnetic resonance imaging (MRI) using three-dimensional (3D) imaging.[3] The germinal matrix releases as many as 100,000 cortical neurons per day, each one migrating through the cortex to its specific predesignated location. Neuronal maturation and organization occurs predominantly around 24 weeks. In the preterm infant, this evolution occurs in the extrauterine life, instead of the intrauterine environment. Hence, this is the period in the NICU, where the brain is most vulnerable to any kind of insult, considering that the preterm baby usually spends a long time in this environment.

At a time when their brain is growing most rapidly, the fetus is suddenly thrown into the chaotic environment of the NICU. In the utero, the fetus is lying in the warm, dark, aquatic environment. When it is born, it suddenly finds itself in the cold, dry, noisy, and excessively bright surroundings of the NICU. However, this "foreign" hi-tech environment is essential for its survival. So, we have to try and understand the neurodevelopmental expectations of this so called "fetal infant" **(Fig. 1)**. Hence, we need to do modification of some NICU practices which are injurious to the developing brain.

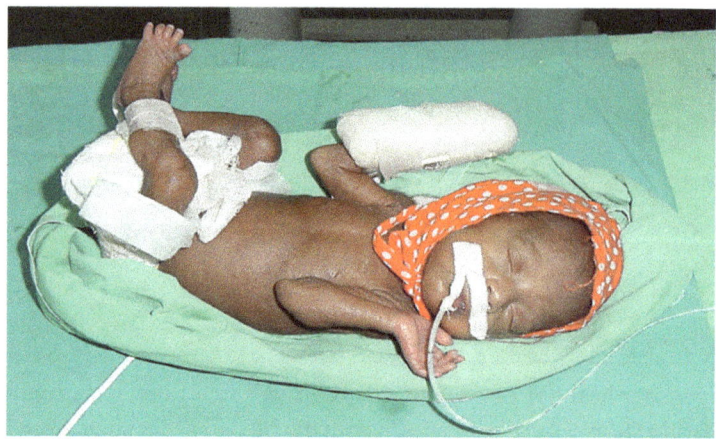

Fig. 1: Nesting.

NOISE

Loud talking, banging of incubator doors, and alarms make the NICU a very noisy place. These loud noises may cause sensorineural hearing loss in preterm babies. Lasky et al.[4] reported 4–13% sensorineural hearing loss in preterm babies depending on their gestation as compared to 2% in all newborns. The US Environment Protection Agency (EPA) has recommended that the ideal sound level should be <45 dB.[5] However, the noise level in our incubators was 50–80 dB and was much higher in the open beds. This high noise level results in increased heart rate, alterations in blood pressure, and consequently decreased cerebral blood flow. The Bengaluru group[6] has developed a low-cost protocol for reducing noise levels in their ventilator room.

The noise level in NICU can be brought down by promptly attending to and anticipating alarms, gently closing incubator doors, and talking softly during rounds. Teaching residents should not be done next to a patient during rounds.

A study from UK[7] showed that the noise level in their transport ambulance on country roads was 120 dB. It is frightening to imagine the noise levels in our ambulance on the pothole-ridden rural roads, especially after the rainy season!

LIGHT

Preterm babies are exposed to the harsh, bright light of the NICU, in stark contrast to the darkness in utero. Reduced light may result in improved sleep cycles and result in decreased stress. Direct light should be avoided as far as possible, unless needed for a procedure. Light can be reduced by putting blankets on the incubator **(Fig. 2)**. Lights can be dimmed to simulate "sleep" time.

PAIN

Many painful procedures are done in the NICU, the heel prick being the most frequently done procedure. The heart rate and oxygen saturation decrease

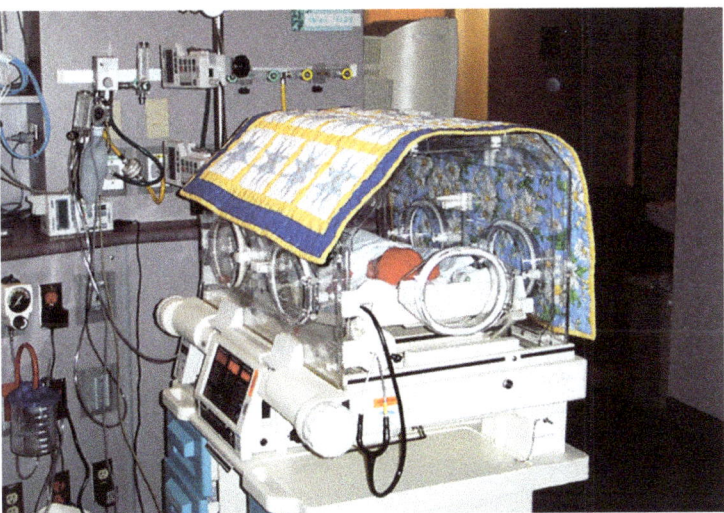

Fig. 2: Covering the incubator to reduce exposure to noise and light.

during the heel prick. The infant gives us clues of pain by grimace, frown, grunting, arching, and recoiling of arms and leg extension. Repetitive pain may cause damage to the developing neurons. This may cause distinct behavioral patterns characterized by anxiety, altered pain and sensitivity to pain, and stress disorders, and this may lead to attention deficit disorders (ADDs).[8]

If clustered care in the form of measuring temperature, changing diapers, mouth care, measuring abdominal girth is done after a painful procedure, such as heel prick, the baby reacts by heightened body, facial, and heart rate responses.[9] Cuddling the baby after a painful procedure is recommended.

TACTILE STIMULI

Routine caregiving activities in the NICU may produce stress in the infant.[8] It may lead to aversive behavior and the baby may associate all touch with pain, which is manifested by squirming, crying, and splaying of arms and legs (**Fig. 3**). Gentle handling, talking softly, and avoiding sudden changes in posture will prevent the fear of tactile stimulation.[9]

MEDICATIONS

Exposure to dexamethasone in this period is neurotoxic to the developing brain. A higher incidence of cerebral palsy (49 vs. 15%) has been reported in babies treated with this drug in a 3-day early trial. 3D MRI images of infants treated with dexamethasone showed impaired growth of cerebral gray matter and a 30% reduction in the total cerebral tissue volume, as compared to controls.[10]

Aminoglycosides and frusemide are known to cause hearing impairment. Benzyl alcohol found in drugs such as midazolam and lorazepam is known to cause cerebral palsy.

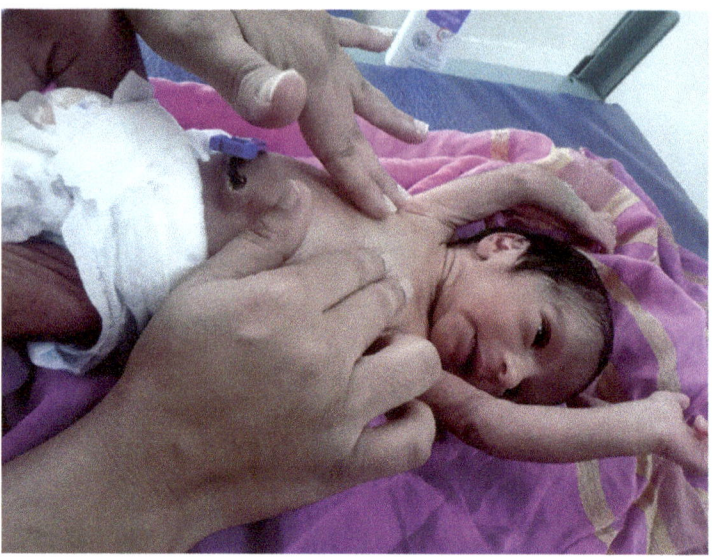

Fig. 3: Splaying of arms following tactile stimulation.

RADIATION

An ELBW baby who is ventilated gets innumerable chest X-rays. Exposure to radiation has been reported to give mental retardation since radiation is known to modify cells. Computed tomography (CT) scans give a much higher dose of radiation. But fortunately, we can now get head MRIs without any radiation.

DEVELOPMENTALLY SUPPORTIVE HUMANIZED CARE

There is a lot of sensory overload in the NICU, a total contrast to the expectations of the developing brain. So, developmentally supportive care aims at creating a "womb out of womb," so that the stress of the infant in the NICU is reduced. The Neonatal Individualized Developmental Care and Assessment Programme (NIDCAP) lays great emphasis on developmental care.[11]

Kangaroo mother care, nesting (*See* **Fig. 1**), soft music, gentle oil massage, swaddling, and cuddling the baby certainly decrease the stress of the baby. Opioids can be used for decreasing pain after operative procedures. Local anesthetic creams containing lidocaine and prilocaine can be used after heel pricks and venipunctures. Paracetamol does not reduce pain after a heel prick, but is used to reduce pain after circumcision. A small amount of dextrose/sucrose can be given during a painful procedure.

For developmentally supportive care, the noise level in the NICU can be brought down. Excessive illumination in the NICU can be reduced. The use of blankets over the incubators can effectively muffle the noise as well as reduce the light. Gentle handling and avoiding sudden changes in posture will help in preventing the fear of the tactile stimulus. It is better to limit the use of steroids in the ELBW infants. Ultrasonography (USG) and MRI are safer modalities for evaluation of the brain.

A developmentally supportive care, which is gentle and sensitive, will certainly enhance the developmental outcome of the preterm infants.

REFERENCES

1. Wilson-Costello D, Friedman H, Munich N, Fanaroff A, Hack M. Improved survival rates with increased neurodevelopmental disability for extremely low birth weight infants. Pediatrics. 2005;115(4):997-1003.
2. Gressens P, Rogida A, Pendaveine B, Sola A. The impact of neonatal intensive care practices on the developing brain. J Pediatr. 2002;140(6):646-52.
3. Counsell SI, Rutherford MA, Cawan FM, Edwards AD. Magnetic resonance imaging of preterm brain injury. Arch Dis Child Fetal Neonatal Ed. 2003;88(4):269-74.
4. Lasky RE, Williams AL. Noise and light exposure for extremely low birth weight newborns during their stay in the neonatal intensive care unit. Pediatrics. 2009;123(2):540-6.
5. Environment Protection Agency. Information on levels of environmental noise requisite to protect public health and welfare with an adequate margin of safety (Report No.5509-74-004). Washington DC: Government Printing Office; 1974.
6. Ramesh A, Rao S, Sandeep G, Nagpoornima M, Srilakshmi V, Dominic M, et al. Efficacy of low cost protocol in reducing noise levels in the neonatal intensive care unit. Indian J Pediatr. 2009;76(5):33-6.
7. Buckland L, Austin N, Jackson A, Inder T. Excessive exposure of sick neonates to sound during transport. Arch Dis Child Fetal Neonatal Ed. 2003;88(6):F513-6.
8. Klein VC, Gaspardo CM, Martinez FE, Grunaun RE, Linhares MB. Pain and distress reactivity and recovery as early predictors of temperament in toddlers born preterm. Early Hum Dev. 2009;85(9):569-76.
9. Holsti L, Grunau RE, Oberland TF, Whitfield MF. Prior pain induces heightened motor responses during clustered care in preterm infants in the NICU. Early Hum Dev. 2005;81(3):293-302.
10. Murphy BP, Inder TE, Huppi PS, Warfield S, Zientara GP, Kikinis R, et al. Impaired cerebral cortical gray matter: growth after treatment with dexamethasone for neonatal chronic lung disease. Pediatrics. 2001;107(2):217-21.
11. Als H, Gilkerson L, Duffy H, McAnulty GB, Beuhler GB, Vandenberg K, et al. A three-center randomized, controlled trial of individualized developmental care for very low birth preterm infants: medical neurodevelopmental, parenting and care giving effects. J Dev Behav Pediatr. 2003;24(6):399-408.

CHAPTER 2

Discharge Planning and Counseling

Sudha Chaudhari

INTRODUCTION

The admission of the newborn to the neonatal intensive care unit (NICU) is not only a stressful but also a scary experience for the parents. They have dreamt of a healthy, bonny baby. Instead they have a sick, scrawny baby to deal with. Their own feelings of guilt and helplessness are compounded by the fact that they have no role to play in the care of the baby, the care is taken over by nurses and doctors.[1] Hence, the professional team needs to give moral support to the parents and guide them on how to manage the baby after discharge at home. The discharge of the sick neonate is the end of a long struggle for both the parents and the baby. Here are a few guidelines while planning the discharge.

PLANNING THE DISCHARGE

The baby should be absolutely stable before planning a discharge. Babies who are born very low birth weight (VLBW) or extremely low birth weight (ELBW) represent an "at risk" group of infants.[1,2] The prerequisites for planning a discharge for these babies are as follows:

- The baby should not require oxygen.
- There should be no apneic spells for 7 days.
- The baby should have recovered from all acute illnesses.
- The baby should be on "katori spoon" and/or partial breastfeeds.
- The baby should be able to maintain his or her temperature of >36°C in a normal household environmental temperature. This is particularly important in the winter season.

The mother is not confident about handling the baby. The baby may have been in the NICU for 6-8 weeks and the nurses have been taking care of the baby. Hence the baby should be transferred to a "step down" unit where the mothers "room in" with the baby and care for the baby with minimal supervision by the nurse.

The prerequisites for the family are as follows:

- The mother should be confident about the feeding technique (breast or katori spoon) and preparing formula feeds if a formula is needed.
- Parents should be happy to take the baby home and should have demonstrated adequate parenting skills.

brainstem evoked response audiometry (BERA) is done to confirm that hearing is normal.

Neurodevelopmental Assessment

This assessment helps to identify early developmental delay. The "High Risk" infant, after the general checkup and neurological examination by the neonatologist, is referred to the occupational therapist who attends the High-risk Clinic.

The therapist assesses the baby at 3, 6, 9, and 12 months corrected age. If there is delay, we give a special stimulation kit (*See* **Chapter 8A**). She instructs the parents about correct carrying positions, advantages of "tummy time", etc.

Development Quotient

The parents are advised to bring the child at 18 months (corrected age) for a development quotient (DQ). This gives a mental and a motor age. The parents are explained that if the DQ is normal and the child is walking, the development is on the right track and they should stop worrying about the child. This relieves a great deal of anxiety in the parents.

Retinopathy of Prematurity

If the preterm baby has ROP, frequent checkups as advised by the ophthalmologist should be done.

The parent guidance book, which we give every mother, lists some (1) practices to be avoided (2) danger signs, and (3) appointments for follow-up.

Practices to be Avoided

- Do not worry; your baby can feel your emotions.
- Do not allow your baby to be touched by unclean hands and use unclean toys.
- Do not stop medication without consulting your doctor.
- Do not supplement breast milk with anything else without consent from your doctor.
- Do not restrict your child from trying new skills.
- Do not make the baby stand till he/she is ready and avoid walkers.

Follow-up Schedule

Name	
Date of birth	
Gestational age	
Corrected date	
Birth weight	
Registration no	
Date of admission	
Date of discharge	

Contd...

Contd...

BERA appointment
(3 months corrected age)

First neurodevelopmental assessment
(3 months corrected age)

Second neurodevelopmental assessment
(6 months corrected age)

Third neurodevelopmental assessment
(9 months corrected age)

Fourth neurodevelopmental assessment
(12 months corrected age)

Developmental quotient (DQ)
(18 months)

Contact Information
For Appointments and Assessments

Contact Persons	Mobile no
Medical Officer	
NICU Coordinator	
Lactation Consultant	
Medical Emergencies	

FREQUENTLY ASKED QUESTIONS

- Which date should we give for the horoscope?
  - Corrected date or birth date?
  - When should we celebrate the baby's birthday?
  - Which date for school admission?
- When do we start breastfeeding?
- How long do we continue KMC?
- When do we start immunization?
- How much weight should a preterm gain per day?
- Should we use air conditioners in summer and heaters in winter?

REFERENCES

1. Tagare A, Chaudhari S, Kadam S, Vaidya UV, Pandit A, Sayyad MG. Mortality and morbidity in extremely low birth (ELBW) infants in neonatal intensive care unit. Indian J Pediatr. 2013;80(1):16-20.
2. Rennie J. Rennie and Robertson's Textbook of Neonatology, 5th edition. London, Elsevier; 2012. pp. 128-32.
3. Chaudhari S, Kulkarni S, Pandit A, Deshmukh S. Mortality and morbidity in high risk infants during a six year follow up. Indian Pediatr. 2000;37(12):1314-20.
4. Nair MKC, Jain N, Murki S, Parthasarathy A. The high risk newborn. New Delhi: Jaypee Brothers Medical Publishers; 2008. pp. 267-9.
5. Filippa M, Lordier L, De Armeida JS, Monaci MG, Adam-Darque A, Grandjean D, et al. Early vocal contact and music in the NICU: new insights into preventive interventions. Pediatr Res. 2020;87(2):249-64.
6. Polkki T, Korhonen A. The effectiveness of music on pain among preterm infants in neonatal intensive care unit: a systematic review. JBI Libr Syst Rev. 2012;10(58):4600-9.

Organization of the High-risk Clinic

CHAPTER

Sudha Chaudhari

INTRODUCTION

The high-risk infant has many problems after discharge. They need close monitoring so that early intervention can be started. These babies cannot be seen in a busy well baby clinic or pediatric outpatient department (OPD), because they need special attention and the services of a multidisciplinary team who can handle their individual needs and spare a little extra time for counseling the parents. Each member of the team needs to be empathetic and patient, because the parents have many anxieties and fears about their precious, fragile infant. If they are seen in the "well baby clinic," unnecessary comparisons will be made with healthy, robust babies and the parents may get depressed.

PATIENT SELECTION

Ideally, all neonatal intensive care unit (NICU) graduates should be seen in this clinic. However, selection can be modified by the strength of the staff and time constraints and overcrowding should be avoided. So, some of the bigger babies, who are stable, can be transferred to the "Well Baby Clinic."

CRITERIA FOR CLOSE MONITORING

- All babies weighing <1,500 g at birth
- All babies with gestational age <36 weeks
- Birth asphyxia resulting in hypoxic ischemic encephalopathy
- Intraventricular hemorrhage grades II, III, and IV
- Septicemia/meningitis
- Hyperbilirubinemia needing exchange transfusion
- All babies who have received ventilatory support
- Symptomatic hypoglycemia
- Seizures other than hypocalcemic seizures
- *Congenital defects:*
  – Chromosomal defects
  – Cardiac problems
  – Operated surgical anomalies such as tracheoesophageal fistula, diaphragmatic hernia, intestinal atresia
- Complex sociofamilial situation

The high-risk infants face many problems after discharge.
- *High postneonatal mortality and morbidity:*
  - In a follow-up study by Chaudhari et al.,[1] out of 404 high-risk infants, 40 deaths (9.4%) occurred in the first year of life, whereas there were no deaths (0%) in 86 full term controls who were being followed up at the same time. Most deaths were due to infections and mortality was highest in the very low birth weight (VLBW) infants.
  - *High morbidity:* These infants also had a high morbidity. 95 infants (23%) had 144 admissions to the hospital. The most common cause was infection and anemia, particularly so in babies from the low socioeconomic class.[1]
  - *Mortality in intervention and nonintervention group:* Out of a total 346 LBW infants who were being followed up regularly, 22 infants died (6.4%). Out of the 58 defaulters, who did not attend the High-risk Clinic (HRC), the mortality rate was 27.6% and this difference was significant. This study[1] emphasizes the importance of a regular follow-up in the HRC.
- *Growth retardation:* The small for gestational age (SGA) infants remained significantly shorter than appropriate for gestational age (AGA) infants and controls. They did not catch up even at the age of 18 years.[2]
- *Neurodevelopmental Handicaps:* The most dreaded sequelae in high-risk infants are cerebral palsy and mental retardation. In a cohort of 404 high-risk infants, cerebral palsy was present in 4% and mental retardation was present in 5% infants and seizure disorder was diagnosed in 3.9%. Hearing impairment was diagnosed in 1.5%.[3] Retinopathy of prematurity (ROP) was found in 22.5% of VLBW infants,[4] and these needed close follow-up in the HRC.

FUNCTIONS AND GOALS OF THE HIGH-RISK CLINIC (FLOWCHART 1)

Primary care should be available round the clock for emergencies. The high-risk card should immediately ensure prompt treatment by the resident doctor.
- Anticipatory guidance regarding growth and development. The concept of corrected age should be explained to the parents of preterm infants. Corrected date should be written on the discharge card.
- Treatment of illnesses
- Immunization

INTERVENTIONS

- *Stimulation*:
  - A simple stimulation program should be given to parents to enhance development.
  - A mobile should be hung over the cradle.
  - A red ball should be moved from side to side when the baby is awake to stimulate vision.

Flowchart 1: The flow of patients in the high-risk clinic.

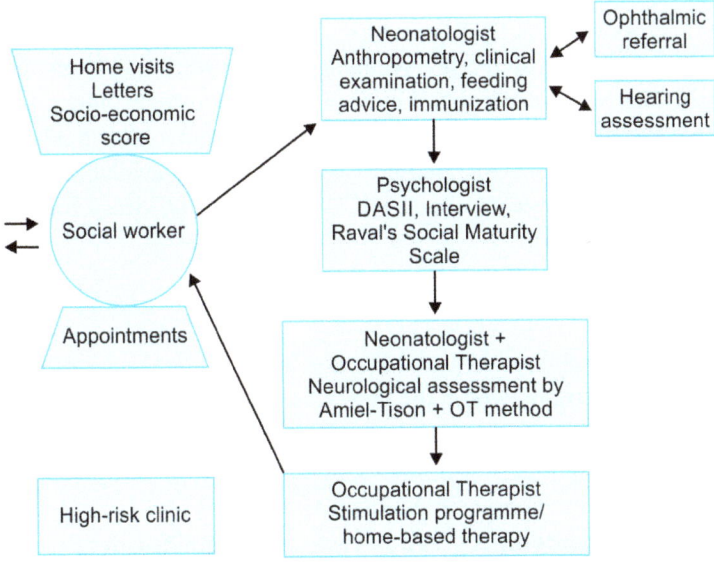

(DASII: developmental assessment scale for Indian infants)

- A "pooja bell" or a rattle should be rung from side to side to stimulate hearing.
- Soft music should be played whenever the baby wakes up for a feed.
- *Remedial therapy*: Infants who show delayed development or tone abnormalities should be referred to the occupational therapist.

ASSESSMENTS

- *Growth and nutrition (Anthropometry):* Growth monitoring is very important especially in our country where a large percentage of high-risk babies are SGA.
- *Neurodevelopmental assessment* should be longitudinal. Early intervention can be started if neurodevelopmental abnormalities are detected. The Amiel-Tison method is a good test to detect tone abnormalities. Many of the maneuvers are common with the Bobath method used by the occupational therapist. So, we have devised a common ATOT form,[3] where the neonatologist and occupational therapist assess the baby together **(Annexure II)**. This cuts down on the duplication of effort and saves a lot of time.
- *Neurosensory* assessment of vision and hearing. Hearing should be assessed at corrected age of 3 months in preterms. Babies who had ROP should be referred to the ophthalmologist.
- *Investigations*: Hemoglobin, metabolic screening, if indicated
- *Imaging* whenever indicated, especially sonography of the brain in infants with intraventricular hemorrhage, or hydrocephalus. Magnetic resonance imaging (MRI) whenever indicated
- *Electroencephalogram (EEG)* for children with seizures

REFERRAL TO OTHER SERVICES

Other services such as ENT (ear, nose, and throat), ophthalmology, and neurosurgery should be readily available without having to travel to other hospitals. The high postneonatal mortality can be brought down if prompt treatment for infections which may result in septicemia, is available. Hence, facilities for readmission to a pediatric ward should be available, if possible under the same physician. Each NICU must have all these facilities for continuity of treatment.

STAFF REQUIREMENTS

The ideal core team should consist of:
- Neonatologist under whom the baby was admitted in the NICU
- A nurse to take anthropometry, give advice regarding feeding. She is an important person for preventing lactation failure. She also gives guidance regarding immunization and family planning.
- Occupational therapist who detects development delay and tone abnormalities and gives therapy, usually a home training program, unless the delay is severe.
- Ideally, a developmental psychologist who can administer developmental tests at 18–24 months.
- *Social worker*: Very important member of the team, who has a close rapport with the family and looks after the human aspect of the family. He allays their fears and anxieties. He gives appointments, sends letters. Makes a home visit if appointments are missed.

Depending on the strength of the NICU, the HRC can be held twice or thrice a week. The doctor attending the HRC must be well-versed with the special needs of these babies such as feeding difficulties, growth rates, nutritional needs, and developmental aberrations. The whole team must provide a unified interdisciplinary approach, so that the mother feels that the entire team is working towards the welfare of her child.

HOW TO CUT COSTS?

- A nurse can be borrowed from the NICU for 2 hours.
- The neonatologist from the NICU can attend the clinic.
- In case there is no funding for a developmental psychologist, the doctor can train himself in some standardized tests such as Amiel-Tison and refer selected cases elsewhere for psychometric evaluation.
- The occupational therapist can design a home-based program, which the parents are taught. The father can shoot a video on his phone while the therapist is teaching the exercises and the baby can be called to the hospital only once a month (Chapters 8A and 8B).
- The social worker can mobilize financial assistance for poor families through voluntary organizations.

EARLY INTERVENTION

The main aim of follow-up services is to identify delayed or abnormal development, so that early intervention can be started (*See* **Chapter 8A**). Ideally, all babies discharged from the NICU need some form of special care. This may be in the form of a special stimulation program or in babies with delayed development, a special remedial program (*See* **Chapter 8B**). Babies found to have auditory impairment, a special oral-aural intervention program will have to be designed with the aid of a hearing aid. In those with profound hearing loss, a cochlear implant may be necessary (*See* **Chapter 4B**).

SCHEDULE OF VISITS

The schedule and frequency of visits will have to be individualized according to the birth weight and other risks and problems. Intense monitoring should be done in the first 3 months and it can be relaxed gradually. The clinic should be held in the afternoon when mothers are comparatively free from housework. All assessments are carried out by predetermined appointments. Developmental tests and neurosensory evaluation is done depending on the facilities available in the hospital. The occupational therapist can do a screening test for tone abnormalities and start a therapy program. The psychologist can assess the mental and motor development by the Developmental Assessment Scales for Indian Infants (DASII) at 18 months corrected age.

Neurosensory evaluation is done by referring the baby to an ophthalmologist for fundoscopy and retinoscopy, especially if the baby was found to have ROP in the NICU.[3] Monthly checkups for ROP till the age of 6 months and subsequently at 1 and 5 years to look for squints and myopias (*See* **Chapter 5A**). Hearing is assessed by Brainstem Evoked Auditory Response audiometry at corrected age of 3 months. Hearing must be assessed again at 3 years by pure tone audiometry to detect hearing loss as this may affect school performance. Three ages are most important in the follow-up of the high-risk infant: 3 months to find out if the baby needs early intervention; 12 months to see how effective the early intervention has been;[3] 4–5 years to detect cognitive problems.

Schedule of visits is shown in **Table 1**.

RECORDKEEPING

A special high-risk card must be designed with a color that is different from the Well Baby Card, so that the baby can be identified as a very important person (VIP) in the emergency room and given prompt treatment. This kind of treatment to the family ensures a good follow-up. The card should have the chronological birth date and the "corrected" birth date in preterms. Telephone numbers of the lactation consultants, emergency nos. and nos., for taking various appointments should be given on the back of the card. The card should be designed on a glossy paper since this ensures that it will last long and will be durable. Each child should have an independent file with the same HRC number on the card and the file.

Organization of the High-risk Clinic

TABLE 1: High-risk clinic: Guidelines for schedule of visits.

Preschedule	Age in months											
	1	2	3	4	5	6	9	12	18	24	36
History, examination, guidance, anthropometry	All visits											
Developmental tests		*				*	*	*	*			
Visual testing	As indicated											
Auditory			*					*				*
Hemogram												
Immunization	As indicated											
Stimulation program	All visits											
Therapy	As indicated											

* Scheduled visit

The first page will have all the clinical data from the NICU. The risk factors can be numbered to facilitate entry in the computer. The second sheet will contain all the details of the visit, such as anthropometry, intercurrent illnesses, treatment, and referrals. The next sheet will have the social worker's interview regarding parents' education, housing, socioeconomic status. A growth chart will be the next sheet. The last sheets are for the assessments of the occupational therapist, psychologist, BERA reports, etc.

The success of a good follow-up program will depend on the cooperation of the parents and their ability to understand the importance of these visits. Many factors such as high travel costs, ignorance, dominance of the mother-in-law, and transfer to other cities are some of the causes for the attrition. The rapport established by the core team, especially by the social worker, will help in a good follow-up. Letters can be sent to the defaulters as reminders, and a home visit can be made by the social worker to find out the cause. It would be ideal if the social worker can make a home visit before discharge, to help organization of the care of the baby at home. This will boost the confidence of the parents in themselves as well as the "high-risk" team and hopefully minimize the drop-out rate.

IS THE EXPENSE JUSTIFIED?

The whole purpose of an expensive hi-tech NICU is defeated if there is no follow-up service. Costs can be cut down by employing a part-time psychologist and therapist. However, the most important member is the social worker, who has to be full time. Some provision has to be made for his travel costs. All this organization needs a lot of administrative backup. Yet, it is absolutely imperative, so that these small, fragile NICU survivors of expensive intensive neonatal care achieve their maximum potential. Cost effectiveness for such a humanitarian service cannot be judged objectively, for it is a fight to improve their quality of life.[1]

REFERENCES

1. Chaudhari S, Kulkarni S, Pandit A, Deshmukh S. Mortality and morbidity in high risk infants during a six year follow up. Indian Pediatr. 2000;37(12):1314-20.
2. Chaudhari S, Otiv M, Khairnar B, Pandit A, Hoge M, Sayyad M. Pune low birth weight study—growth from birth to adulthood. Indian Pediatr 2012;49(9):727-32.
3. Chaudhari S, Kulkarni S, Barve S, Pandit A, Sonak U, Sarpotdar N. Neurologic sequelae in high risk infants: a three year follow up. Indian Pediatr. 1996;33(8):645-53.
4. Chaudhari S, Patwardhan V, Vaidya U, Kadam S, Kamat A. Retinopathy of prematurity in a tertiary care center: incidence, risk factors and outcome. Indian Pediatr. 2009;46(3):219-24.

CHAPTER 4A

Hearing Assessment in Infants

Neelam Vaid, Shweta Deshpande

INTRODUCTION

Hearing loss in neonates and infants is not easy to identify either by routine clinical examination or behavioral observation. It is, therefore, commonly referred to as an invisible disability.

Hearing loss is the most common sensory disability at birth. According to World Health Organization (WHO) (2018),[1] around 466 million people worldwide have disabling hearing loss, and 34 million of these are children. About 63 million people are estimated to have significant hearing loss in India and the incidence of childhood-onset deafness is 2%. Early-onset hearing loss in India is about 5–6 per 1,000 live births, making it even more than congenital hypothyroidism and phenylketonuria. It is estimated that about 30,000 children are born every year, with some degree of hearing impairment. Even more will develop hearing loss during childhood.

THE HEARING BRAIN

Hearing is a sensory function and more of a passive process, whereas listening is an active process requiring the brain to attend and react accordingly. The hearing brain involves about 100 billion nerve cells and 1,015 connections. The child's brain is preconditioned to accept and process sound. The development of listening skills is influenced by auditory stimulation at a critical age and genetic factors. Exposure to meaningful sounds is essential for the development of the auditory pathways and auditory cortex, which begins in the intrauterine phase at about 20 weeks of gestation. By the time a baby is born with hearing loss, the development of the auditory pathway is already set back by about 20 weeks. If a baby does not receive auditory stimulation during the early years, then the nerve cells and their connections, through a process of synaptic pruning, will result in enhanced processing through other senses, primarily vision in this case, also described as cross-modal plasticity.[2,3]

Hearing loss in childhood affects the development of speech and language acquisition, which in turn affects literacy, leading to fewer employment opportunities. It is estimated that 90% of a young child's knowledge is attributed to incidental reception of sounds; this learning is affected with even the slightest hearing loss. Hart and Risley[3] demonstrated that the number of words heard by a child affects their vocabulary and intelligence quotient (IQ). Children who heard ~30,100 words in a 14-hour day had a vocabulary of

~1,100 words and an IQ of 117 at age 3 years, while children who heard ~8,600 words in a day had a vocabulary of 525 words and an IQ of 79. Early hearing deprivation could affect not only language but also cognitive functions, such as decreased executive function, disturbed personality, abnormal social behavior, and delayed decision-making and enhanced visual attention.[4,5] An inability to communicate affects the development of social skills and leads to anger, frustration, and loneliness in the child. All this has a profound effect on the family and caregivers. Even children with mild sensorineural loss or single-sided deafness experience challenges in school and psychosocial issues.

It has been shown both in animal models and children that the first 3 years of life are critical for maturation of the auditory cortex.[6] Insufficient or no stimulation of the auditory cortex during the sensitive periods of plasticity could lead to abnormality of auditory and language development. The most critical period for the development of speech and language is the first 3 years of life. After this, the brain has reduced plasticity to process auditory information. Timing, therefore, is critical to optimize outcomes.

CAUSES OF HEARING LOSS IN INFANTS

Hearing loss in these children could be congenital, i.e., present at birth or acquired in which the causative factor occurs later.

Congenital

All patients with congenital hearing loss are prelingual, i.e., their hearing loss has occurred before the development of speech and language, and this has a major effect on their communication and academic development. Hearing loss present at birth could be due to the following reasons:
- *Genetic*: 50% of congenital hearing loss is transmitted by a genetic code. 70% of these are nonsyndromic and 30% are syndromic.
  - *Nonsyndromic*: Autosomal recessive inheritance accounts for 80%, autosomal dominant about 19%, and <1% are due to mitochondrial and X-linked genes.
  - *Syndromic*: Numerous syndromes are associated with hearing impairment.
- *Factors that interfere with embryological development*: Maternal infections are the main offenders in this subset. 16 viruses and 6 bacteria can adversely affect the fetus, the common ones are TORCH (toxoplasmosis, others, rubella, cytomegalovirus, herpes) or STORCH (includes syphilis) and recently, the ZIKA virus. Cytomegalovirus (CMV) is the most common viral cause of congenital hearing loss. 85% of children with hearing impairment due to CMV have severe-to-profound hearing loss, and 50% have at least one additional disability.[7]
  - Ototoxic medication, such as aminoglycosides, given to the mother during the antenatal period can cause hearing impairment.
  - Other antenatal factors such as maternal diseases like diabetes and nutritional deficiencies can contribute to hearing impairment.

- *Factors that occur during the birth process*: Perinatal prolonged labor and trauma during labor can cause hearing loss. Borg[7] reviewed the relationship between hearing loss and perinatal hypoxia, ischemia, and asphyxia. The risk of permanent hearing loss was more with ischemia than hypoxia. Kumar K et al.[8] found that the incidence of hearing impairment in infants with hypoxic ischemic encephalopathy was about 7%. The incidence of hearing impairment is more in those neonates that required assisted ventilation. 4% of infants with hyperbilirubinemia are likely to have hearing impairment.

Acquired

Otitis media, administration of ototoxic drugs, especially aminoglycoside antibiotics, meningitis, and encephalitis, are common causes of acquired hearing impairment. The presence of risk factors such as prematurity, hyperbilirubinemia, administration of ototoxic drugs, and hypoxia increase the likelihood of developing auditory neuropathy spectrum disorder (ANSD).

Table 1 lists the risk factors commonly associated with hearing loss (JCIH 2019).[9]

HEARING ASSESSMENT

As timing is of critical value in the diagnosis of hearing impairment, it is advocated that early detection via neonatal hearing screening is conducted on all babies.[10] Hearing screening, followed by a detailed diagnostic audiological evaluation and intervention, will lay the foundation for spoken language development.

Newborn Hearing Screening[11]

The aim of any hearing screening program is early detection and intervention (EHDI) to maximize linguistic, communicative competence, and literacy

TABLE 1: Risk indicators for hearing loss (JCIH, 2019).

1.	Family history of hearing loss since childhood
2.	Infants who require NICU admission for >5 days
3.	Hyperbilirubinemia requiring exchange transfusion
4.	Aminoglycoside administration for >5 days
5.	Perinatal asphyxia (hypoxic ischemic encephalopathy), especially if requiring hypothermia treatment
6.	Extracorporeal membrane oxygenation (ECMO)
7.	In utero infections—TORCH and ZIKA virus
8.	Craniofacial and physical abnormalities
9.	Syndromic infants
10.	Perinatal/postnatal confirmed bacterial and/or viral meningitis or encephalitis (especially herpes, varicella, *Haemophilus influenzae*, and pneumococcal)
11.	Postnatal events such as head injury or receiving chemotherapy
12.	Family/caregiver concerns regarding hearing or speech and language development

(NICU: neonatal intensive care unit; TORCH: toxoplasmosis, others, rubella, cytomegalovirus, herpes)

development in children who have a hearing impairment. These were not detected till 2-3 years of age, and those with hearing thresholds between 25 and 40 dB were not detected till school age.[11] However, Holte et al. showed that the average age of diagnosis and age of referral for early intervention have steadily decreased over the years.

There are three types of population-based screening programs.
1. *Universal*: Every newborn undergoes a hearing screening.
2. *Risk factor*: Only babies with a risk factor underwent screening for hearing impairment. This screening technique can miss 50% of neonates with hearing impairment.
3. *Opportunistic*: Screening is done when a parent/caregiver voiced concerns about the child's hearing.

Wake et al.,[10] in their study, found that the average age of diagnosis with universal screening was 8.1 months, risk factor screening was 16.2 months, and opportunistic screening was 22.5 months.

Timing of Screening

The Joint Committee of Infant Hearing (2007)[11] recommends an ideal EHDI program with a 1-3-6 goal **(Table 2)**. Hearing screening for newborns in well baby nurseries is done close to hospital discharge but before 1 month of age.[12] **Flowchart 1** outlines the recommended schedule for screening well babies.

Screening for the neonatal intensive care unit (NICU) newborn is done when they are ready for discharge or/when they are medically stable. **Flowchart 2** outlines the screening schedule for NICU graduates. Due to the high-risk of auditory neuropathy and hearing impairment, it is preferable to screen these infants with automated auditory behavioral response (AABR) than

TABLE 2: Early hearing detection and intervention.

1.	All infants should undergo hearing screening prior to discharge from the birth hospital and no later than 1 month of age, using physiologic measures with objective determination of outcome
2.	All infants whose initial birth screen and any subsequent rescreening warrant additional testing should have appropriate audiologic evaluation to confirm the infant's hearing status no later than 3 months of age
3.	A concurrent or immediate comprehensive otologic evaluation should occur for infants who are confirmed to be deaf or hard of hearing
4.	All infants who are deaf or hard of hearing in one or both ears should be referred immediately-to-early intervention in order to receive targeted and appropriate services
5.	A simplified, coordinated point of entry into an intervention system appropriate for identified children is optimal
6.	Early intervention services should be offered through an approach that reflects the family's preferences and goals for their child, and should begin as soon as possible after diagnosis but no later than 6 months of age
7.	The child and family should have immediate access, through their audiologist, to high-quality, well-fitted, and optimized hearing aid technology. Access should also be assured, depending on the child's needs, to cochlear implants (CIs), hearing assistive technologies, and visual alerting and informational devices.

Flowchart 1: Hearing screening protocol (well baby clinic).

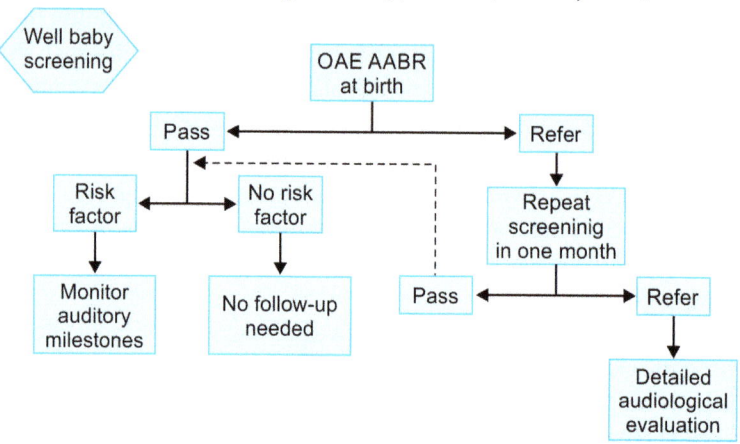

(AABR: automated auditory brainstem response; OAE: otoacoustic auditory emission)

Flowchart 2: Hearing screening protocol [neonatal intensive care unit (NICU)].

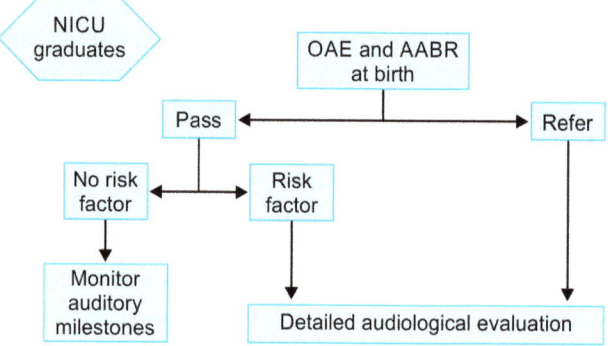

(AABR: automated auditory brainstem response; OAE: otoacoustic auditory emission)

otoacoustic auditory emission (OAE). It is recommended that if screening is done by OAE, a detailed audiological evaluation is advisable irrespective of the screening result. Due to the high incidence of these infants developing hearing loss, they need to be evaluated by an audiologist as soon as possible and closely monitored.[12]

The Joint Committee on Infant Hearing (JCIH) 2019[9] position statement recommends that clinics should set 1-2-3 as a target, especially for those programs who have met the 1-3-6 benchmark (screening completed by 1 month of age, diagnostic evaluation by 2 months, and intervention by 3 months of age).

SCREENING TECHNIQUES

Behavioral Observation

Behavioral observation involves giving a stimulus to the child and looking for a response appropriate to the child's developmental age. The results, however, are highly subjective and, therefore, susceptible to bias. It is also not possible to identify those with mild or moderate hearing impairment or those with unilateral hearing impairment.

Objective Tests for Screening

There are two screening tests, otoacoustic emissions (OAE) and automated auditory brainstem response (AABR) audiometry, used to screen neonates and infants for hearing loss. These tests are noninvasive, easily performed, give information on each ear separately, and do not require any individual's participation. Both OAE and AABR have a high sensitivity for the detection of hearing loss. However, the specificity of OAE is not as high as AABR. AABR can be used to screen for auditory neuropathy for which OAE alone is inappropriate. AABR has a significantly lower refer rate (16.7%) as compared to OAE (37.9%). The referral rates are lowest if the screening is done 48 hours after birth.[12] Unlike behavioral testing, which tests "hearing," these provide information about the integrity of the auditory pathway. However, they require slightly expensive instruments.

Otoacoustic Emissions[3]

Otoacoustic emissions are low-intensity sounds emitted by the outer hair cells of the cochlea. These sounds are measured by inserting a probe in the ear canal and presenting a series of click (acoustic stimulus) sounds to the ear. The presence of OAE picked up by the probe microphone reveals normal functioning by the outer hair cells in the cochlea **(Fig. 1)**. The screening instruments used for testing have transient evoked otoacoustic emission (TEOAE) and distortion product otoacoustic emission (DPOAE) technology. TEOAEs are most often used for newborn infant screening. This test is relatively quick and does not require the placement of any electrodes. The result obtained in the screening test is either pass or refer. It is essential to know that the OAE test does not quantify the hearing loss or assess the integrity of the transmission

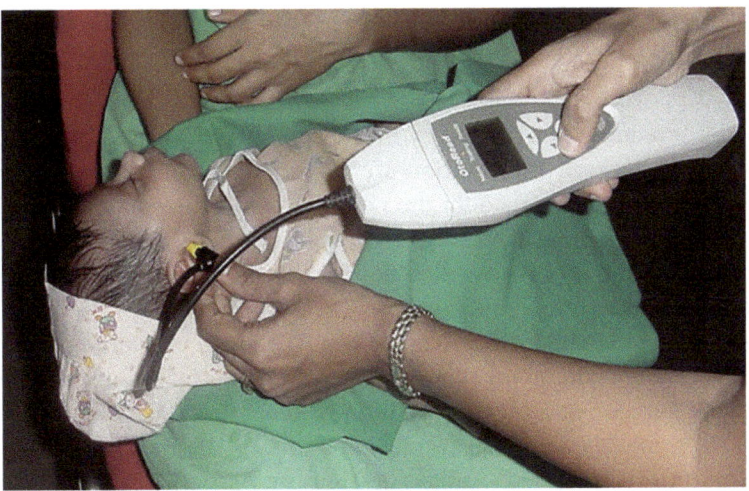

Fig. 1: Otoacoustic emission (OAE).

TABLE 3: Comparison between otoacoustic auditory emission (OAE) and automated auditory behavioral response (AABR) [brainstem evoked response audiometry (BERA)].

	OAE	AABR
Preparation time	No preparation needed	Scrubbing needs to be done for electrode placement
Test time	• Actual test time is about 30 seconds. • Time for test, documentation not more than 10 minutes	• Actual test time is 10 minutes. The entire process can take 20–30 minutes
Referral rate	Higher is comparison to AABR	Low
Cost of disposables	Lesser in comparison to AABR	More than OAE
Susceptibility to outer and middle ear status	Affected by wax, debris, and middle ear fluid	Less affected than OAE
What does the test measure?	The function of the outer hair cells of the cochlea	The auditory pathway
False negatives	• ANSD • Sloping hearing loss	High frequency hearing loss

(ANSD: auditory neuropathy spectrum disorder)

of sound from the auditory nerve to the auditory cortex. A two-stage screening process using both OAE and AABR is considered to be the best method.

Automated Auditory Brainstem Response Audiometry

The AABR screening test uses click stimulus presented at 35–40 dBnHL and detects the summation of action potentials from the auditory nerve to the inferior colliculus in the midbrain. The time needed for screening is 4–15 minutes and requires the placement of electrodes. The test interpretation is done as a pass or fail/refer report. A refer/fail report given by the AABR indicates that the hearing level is worse than 35–40 dB. The test can be done within the first 48 hours after birth. This screening test is much more reliable than OAE.

Table 3 gives a summary of the comparison between these two modalities.

DIAGNOSTIC TESTS FOR HEARING ASSESSMENT[11]

Hearing screening is a necessary first step, but diagnosis, amplification, and referral for early intervention are equally important. The assessment tools should be appropriate for the neurodevelopmental state of the child. A thorough assessment of hearing may require multiple sessions. Thus, serial evaluations may be necessary to develop reliable profiles of hearing status and developmental abilities.

Assessment begins with a detailed history-taking, physical examination of the ears, and taking some time to observe and informally interact with the child and the parents to develop an impression of the child's developmental level. Corrected age should be used in preterms.

The American Speech-Language-Hearing Association (ASHA, 2004) has developed guidelines for assessing the hearing of children from birth through 5 years of age.[13] The aim was to facilitate the hearing evaluation of children who were either identified through screening programs or referred directly to audiologists for hearing assessment and to improve outcomes from early intervention programs. The protocols recommended for children up to 4 months and those with developmental delay and multiple other health issues, use physiologic measures of hearing, i.e., auditory brainstem response (ABR)/auditory steady state response (ASSR), OAE, and acoustic immittance evaluation.

BEHAVIORAL ASSESSMENT

Behavioral Observation Audiometry

Behavioral assessment of hearing in children is complex and influenced by developmental and maturational factors. There is a sequence during development as to when and which sounds babies will respond to. Auditory Behaviour Index summarizes these expected responses during the first two and a half years of life. Behavioral assessment depends on knowing the response appropriate for the child's development.

Behavioral observation audiometry (BOA) is done by presenting sounds using a pediatric audiometer or in the sound field room via loudspeakers. The baby's responses to sounds are observed and recorded by the audiologist. Generally, it is better to involve two examiners, one in the testing room and the other with the baby and the parent. However, due to the high variability in the responses and their detection, a reliable estimation of hearing is not possible. Thus, this test is a corroboration, gives a picture of the development of the child's global auditory behavior rather than an accurate estimation of the hearing impairment.

Visual Reinforcement Audiometry

Visual reinforcement audiometry (VRA) involves the use of conditioned localization response from the child in response to a stimulus along with a visual reinforcer. As the child needs to localize the sound that involves turning the head toward the sound source and the visual reinforcer, this test is appropriate for babies more than 4 months of age. The neuromotor development of the baby by this age permits the head turn response toward the sound source.

This method involves testing in a two-room sound field set-up where the control room has the audiometer with the audiologist and the other room has the loudspeaker and the associated visual reinforcer where the infant and the parent are seated. Depending on the infant's age and developmental level, the baby can be seated in the parent's lap or an infant high chair, facing the table. The second examiner usually distracts the baby with midline distracters, so that they are facing forward. The visual reinforcer is an illuminated toy that moves in its place. When the sound stimulus is presented, the baby is expected to turn his/her head toward the sound and then the reinforcement toy is illuminated. The visual reinforcement with the toy serves as a reward for the baby, thus constituting the conditioning principle. For the response to be acceptable, the baby must demonstrate a clear head turn toward the loudspeaker when they hear the sound. Like in BOA, responses can be judged by two examiners. Thresholds can be determined by using frequency specific stimulus. This procedure is recommended till 2 years of age.[14] Over 2 years of age, the child tends to get habituated more quickly to the stimulus, hence the need for conditioned play audiometry (CPA).

Conditioned Play Audiometry (CPA)

Conditioned play audiometry or play audiometry is most useful for children above 2 years of age up to 5 years of age.[13,14] In this test, the child needs to be trained to respond to auditory stimuli with a specific motor response. For example, the child is trained to hold a block/small toy near the ear and put it in the box/bag once he hears the sound. The testing is done in a two-room set-up as in BOA or VRA. The stimulus is presented through the headphones, insert earphones, or the bone vibrator. In a cooperative child, frequency-specific testing can be done in both the ears to determine the thresholds.

Speech Audiometry

Babies as young as 6 months of developmental age can undergo speech perception or speech audiometry testing. The purpose of testing is to check their ability to perceive speech stimuli. It includes speech awareness, discrimination, and recognition testing. Like in CPA, the stimulus is presented through insert earphones or headphones or loudspeakers. In young babies, speech awareness testing helps correlate the findings along with other behavioral and electrophysiological tests. As the baby grows, developmentally appropriate speech stimulus is used to determine the speech reception threshold.

ELECTROPHYSIOLOGICAL MEASURES

Electrophysiological tests are objective tests wherein the individual's hearing ability is assessed without their active participation or cooperation. These tests provide us with valuable cross-checks on the behavioral results. In infants and young children, these electrophysiological tests dominate in the decision-making process regarding the management of the hearing loss. However, the electrophysiological and behavioral tests provide information on different aspects of the child's auditory function, hence cannot work as substitutes for each other.

Auditory Brainstem Response/Brainstem Evoked Response Audiometry (BERA)[4]

Auditory brainstem response provides diagnostic information about the child's neurological integrity at the brainstem level. The purpose of ABR is to determine the type and severity of hearing loss and provide frequency

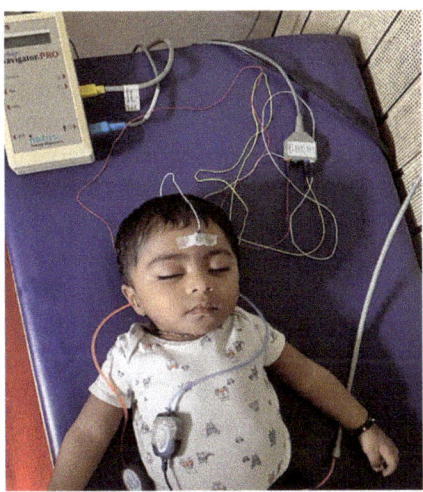

Fig. 2: Brainstem evoked response audiometry (BERA).

specific information. ABR is conducted on newborns, infants, and children of any age, who cannot be assessed by behavioral tests. It is usually done in a quiet or soundproof room. The test requires significant patient preparation, and the child needs to be sleeping during the procedure. Natural sleep is the best, however, if this is not possible, then the child should be sedated. Thus, the testing time is more and might require repeated visits if the child does not sleep. The stimuli used for ABR are the click stimulus, which contains energy over a broad frequency range, i.e., 2,000–4,000 Hz, and the brief duration tone burst stimulus that provides frequency specific information, i.e., 250 Hz or 500 Hz or 1,000 Hz tone bursts **(Fig. 2)**. The stimuli are presented through insert earphones in case of air conduction testing and a standard bone oscillator in case of bone conduction testing. While testing children with external ear or pinna anomalies, supra-aural headphones will be necessary.

Prediction of the audiogram using the ABR is possible. The ABR will be affected by the neurologic status of the child. If the auditory system is damaged and neurons cannot fire synchronously, or if there are disruptions of the auditory pathway due to an insult, there will be no identifiable ABR waveform. Thus, in such cases, the other test findings such as OAE and behavioral test results must be considered before the final diagnosis.

Auditory Steady State Response

Auditory steady state responses are recorded from the scalp and elicited in response to sinusoidal amplitude and frequency-modulated tones.[15] The purpose of ASSR is to estimate the hearing levels at individual frequencies in each ear. This test also requires the child to be sleeping like in ABR.

Acoustic Immittance Evaluation

Acoustic immittance evaluation is an integral part of the test battery that assesses middle ear function and auditory pathway integrity. It is helpful to evaluate the status of the middle ear. It must be performed routinely as a component of the hearing evaluation, and more frequently for children at increased risk for middle ear disease or at risk for auditory neuropathy. Tympanometry and acoustic reflex tests are included in the immittance evaluation. In infants less then 6 months of age, a higher probe tone frequency such as 1,000 Hz has been advocated[14] during testing for identifying middle ear fluid or effusion.[9] Testing is carried out in a quiet area and sedation is not required as it is quickly recorded. However, the babies or children must be resting quietly during the test or they can be distracted by showing a video or pictures. Before testing, it is imperative to perform otoscopy to determine if the external auditory canal is occluded by wax or other debris, as this may affect measurements. Acoustic reflexes help to investigate the possibility of auditory neuropathy when combined with OAE and ABR.

EXCEPTIONAL CONSIDERATIONS/CASES

Newborn hearing screening programs are an excellent initial step to detect hearing loss in infants. However, they are not perfect. There are certain conditions wherein the infants might pass the hearing screening but develop significant permanent hearing loss later. Thus, constant surveillance is needed to detect these infants with hearing loss, who are missed during the screening and begin intervention as soon as possible.[11] These exceptional cases are discussed below.

Mild Hearing Loss or Hearing Loss in Restricted Frequency Regions

Infants with mild hearing loss or specific frequency hearing loss will most often pass newborn hearing screening. In such cases, there is a necessity for a detailed audiological evaluation. The challenge is how to identify these infants. Parents and medical professionals need to be equally aware of auditory and language milestones as they are with other developmental milestones. Any concern raised by the parents regarding the baby's hearing and communication, needs to be addressed immediately.

Fluctuating Hearing Loss Due to Middle Ear Effusion

Otitis media is the most common disease diagnosed in infants and young children which causes fluctuating conductive hearing loss. This type of hearing loss is temporary in nature but, during this time, the child may miss out on the necessary information for speech and language development. If the infection is recurring and chronic, it might cause a permanent sensorineural hearing loss. Thus, immediate attention must be provided by the pediatrician or an otolaryngologist in case of an ear infection. Two additional specialists, i.e., the audiologist and the speech language pathologist, must be involved in case of a recurrent problem.

Auditory Neuropathy Spectrum Disorder

This spectrum encompasses auditory disorders due to abnormalities in the auditory nerve and/or the synapses between the inner hair cells and the auditory nerve. Ten percent of children with sensorineural loss have ANSD. It is seen in up to 10% of well babies and 40% of those from the NICU. A comprehensive medical, developmental, audiological, and communication assessment is recommended for babies suspected with ANSD. The recommended audiological test battery for infants with ANSD, consists of behavioral response to pure tones and speech, measures of middle ear function, tests of cochlear hair cell function, and auditory nerve function. As the outer hair cells are normal in these cases, OAEs are present in a majority of the cases. Frequent audiological evaluation is necessary in infants and young children with ANSD to assess their behavioral responses to sound and auditory development.

We have introduced a universal neonatal hearing screening program at KEM Hospital, Pune, in 2006. The Audiology and Speech Language Therapy unit housed in the TDH. Morris Rehabilitation Centre focuses on early diagnosis and intervention in children with hearing and communication impairment. One of the biggest initial challenges was creating awareness about the importance of hearing screening among the professionals and the parents. We have successfully screened more than 6,000 babies. The screening is done by a paramedic and supervised by an audiologist. Till recently, we were following the 1-3-6 protocol recommended by JCIH. However, now we are performing detailed audiological evaluation in children as early as 1 month. In our center, the incidence of hearing impairment was 5.41/1,000 live births. Follow-up of the families after screening is equally important, as awareness about hearing impairment and its implications are sorely lacking in the general population. In our experience, parents do not realize the impact of hearing loss on speech and language development. As the diagnosis of hearing loss requires a battery of tests and repeated visits, parents hesitate to follow-up in the center and insist on getting the tests done in one visit. They fail to accept that testing babies and young children is not an easy task. After screening and diagnosis, proper counseling regarding the management options and having a team of dedicated professionals is important for successful implementation and intervention. The team in our department is focused on achieving its motto, "Its not just hearing, its about communication."

Audiological assessment consisting of electrophysiologic tests and behavioral observations is necessary in order to expedite the management of children with hearing loss and maximize the opportunity to provide listening during critical period of development. Once the hearing loss is diagnosed, the family's acceptance and readiness to accept the intervention is the next step for achieving good outcome. Intervention with an amplification device, hearing assistive device, and/or cochlear implants along with auditory training should be initiated as soon as possible. Multiple sessions may be required for a complete and thorough assessment. A reliable profile of the hearing status and developmental abilities may require serial evaluations. Finally, the success of any early intervention program lies in the involvement and support of the audiology team.

REFERENCES

1. World Health Organization. (2020). Deafness and hearing loss [online]. Available from: https://www.who.int/news-room/fact-sheets/detail/deafness-and-hearing-loss. [Last accessed January, 2021].
2. Flexer C. Auditory speech and language development. In: Northern JL, Downs MP (Eds). Hearing in Children, 6th edition. San Diego: Plural Publishing; 2014.
3. Hart B, Risley TR. Meaningful differences in the everyday experience of young American children. Baltimore: Paul H Brookes Publishing; 1995.
4. Figueras B, Edwards L, Langdon D. Executive function and language in deaf children. J Deaf Stud Deaf Educ. 2008;13(3):362-77.
5. Kral A, Tillein J, Heid S, Hartmann R, Klinke R. Postnatal cortical development in congenital auditory deprivation. Cereb Cortex. 2005;15(5):552-62.
6. Scildroth AN. Hearing parents' reactions. In: Meadow-Orlans KP, Spencer ES, Koester LS (Eds). The World of Deaf Infants: a longitudinal study, perspectives on deafness. Oxford: Oxford University Press; 2004.
7. Borg E. Perinatal asphyxia, hypoxia, ischemia and hearing loss: an overview. Scand Audiol. 1997;26(2):77-91.
8. Kumar K, Khmour A, Knutson A, Hunter K, Forster L, Kilbride H. Hearing loss in infants with hypoxic-ischemic encephalopathy. Pediatrics. 2018;141(1 Meeting Abstract) 525.
9. Joint Committee on Infant Hearing. Year 2019 Position Statement: Principles and Guidelines for Early Hearing Detection and Intervention Programs. J Early Hear Detect Interv. 2019;4(2):1-44.
10. Wake M, Ching TY, Wirth K, Poulakis Z, Mensah FK, Gold L, et al. Population outcomes of three approaches to detection of congenital hearing loss. Pediatrics. 2016;137(1):e20151722.
11. Joint Committee on Infant Hearing. (2007). Year 2007 Position Statement: Principles and guidelines for early hearing detection and intervention programs. [online] Available from: http://www.jcih.org/posstatemts.htm. [Last accessed January, 2021].
12. VanDyk M, DeWet S, Hall JW. Outcomes with OAE and AABR screening in the first 48h—Implications for newborn hearing screening in developing countries. Int J Pediatr Otorhinolaryngol. 2015;79(7):1034-40.
13. American Speech-Language-Hearing Association. (2004). Guidelines for the Audiologic Assessment of Children From Birth to 5 Years of Age [online]. Available from: www.asha.org/policy. [Last accessed January, 2021].
14. American Academy of Audiology. (2012). Audiologic Guidelines for the Assessment of Hearing in Infants and Young Children. [online] Available from: https://audiologyweb.s3.Amazon aws.com/migrated/201208_AudGuideAssessHear_youth.pdf_5399751b249593.36017703.pdf. [Last accessed January, 2021].
15. Picton TW, John MS, Dimitrijevic A, Purcell D. Human auditory steady-state responses. Int J Audiol. 2003;42(4):177-219.

Intervention in Children with Hearing Loss

CHAPTER 4B

Neelam Vaid, Shweta Deshpande

INTRODUCTION

Early detection, identification, and intervention of hearing loss in infants pave the path for optimal speech, language, and communication development. Once the infant is diagnosed with hearing loss, the onus lies on the audiologist to provide information to the parents and/or the family members regarding the test results and further management options. English[1] has suggested certain guidelines that an audiologist can follow while reporting the child's hearing loss to the parents. It includes aspects such as ensuring privacy, providing adequate time to the parents to understand the child's problem, encouraging them to express their thoughts and feelings, responding to them with warmth and empathy, and respecting the family's decision.

Majority of the children with severe-to-profound hearing loss are born to parents who have normal hearing sensitivity.[2] Thus, they are unaware about the impact of hearing loss on listening skills and spoken language development. Parents react to the diagnosis of hearing loss in different ways. Some have feelings of anger, guilt, disbelief, and detachment, while others readily accept the diagnosis and strive to work towards a solution. It is observed quite often, that parents seek different professional opinions and alternate modes of treatment during this phase. Parents' responses will affect the time taken to seek early intervention services, however it is necessary to provide them with a specific time frame to accept the hearing loss and decide the future action plan. Parental support counseling is not a one-time event but a series of conversations over time by different professionals, especially the pediatrician and the audiologist, regarding the treatment options and long-term rehabilitation plan.[1]

Depending on the etiology and type of hearing loss, the management can be medical/surgical intervention, amplification with hearing aids or implantable hearing devices, and aural rehabilitation.

MEDICAL/SURGICAL INTERVENTION

A comprehensive medical evaluation is necessary by the pediatrician and the otolaryngologist after the hearing loss is identified to determine and identify the cause along with any associated conditions.

Hearing loss due to disorders in the external or middle ear usually respond to medical therapy. In some instances, minor surgical procedures such as removal of wax or insertion of ventilation tubes may be required.

TYPES OF HEARING DEVICES

In children with hearing loss due to abnormalities in the cochlea (sensory), auditory nerve (neural), or the auditory pathway, hearing devices are a proven mode of intervention. The type of device depends on the severity of the hearing loss and the anatomy of the inner ear. Radiological evaluation with respect to temporal bone and brain imaging has gained importance and helped professionals plan the appropriate management option. It has specifically benefitted in identifying anatomical markers for further progression of the loss, deciding appropriate management option with respect to hearing aids or cochlear implants, and predicting prognosis from the hearing devices.[3]

Hearing Aids

A hearing aid is an amplification device designed to make sound more audible to an individual with hearing loss. The common parts of a hearing aid are a microphone to pick up sound, amplifier that makes the sound louder, a receiver that delivers the sound to the ear canal, and batteries to power the electronics (**Fig. 1**). There are many available options which differ in design, the type of amplification (analog or digital), and other special features.

The primary objective of an amplification device is to provide auditory access to the infant or child with hearing loss, with respect to speech and nonspeech sounds occurring in our everyday environment. This will enable the infant/young child to develop optimal communication, literacy, and psychosocial skills.[4] Fitting of a hearing aid involves selection of appropriate hearing aid, making an earmold to link the device with the ear canal, programming and verifying the fitting, and validating the benefit from amplification. Parents of infants with hearing loss must be counseled about hearing aid-fitting process and ongoing hearing assessment. It is necessary to make the family understand that young children cannot provide immediate feedback after the device is fitted, thus careful observation and monitoring of the responses over time is the key to success. Also, the fitting process in children must be conducted by an audiologist who has expertise in pediatric amplification and uses evidence-based protocols.[5]

There are different types of hearing aids (**Fig. 2**). Selection of a specific style will depend on the diagnostic information with respect to the severity and configuration of hearing loss, physical characteristics such as the ear canal size

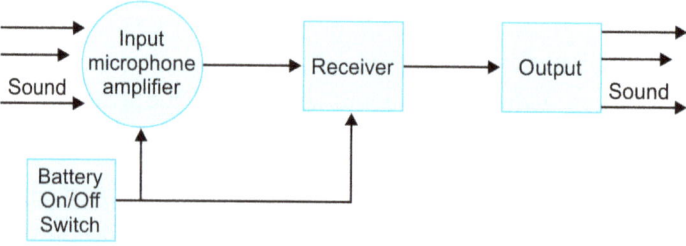

Fig. 1: Simple block diagram of a hearing aid.

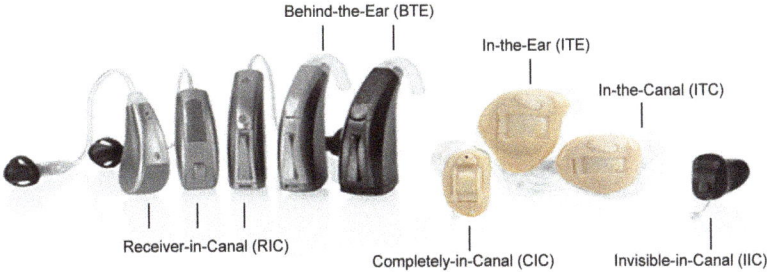

Fig. 2: Types of hearing aids.

and shape, needs of the child, and audiologist's expertise.[4] Infants and young children with severe-to-profound hearing loss are often fitted with bilateral behind-the-ear (BTE) hearing aids. The earmolds in such young children need to be changed frequently, due to changes in the size of their ear canals.

After the device is fitted, the child and the parents are referred to early intervention services as soon as possible. The team comprising of speech language therapists, teachers of the deaf/special educators, and the medical professionals work together with the child and the family. A monthly follow-up schedule is recommended by the team after fitting the aids. It is observed that parents face challenges with respect to the fitting of the earmolds into the ear canal, and increasing the acceptance of the aid by the child. Majority of the parents report that children reject the devices, do not want to wear the aids, or want to take control over it. During this period, they need to be counseled that gradual increase in the use time is beneficial.

Over time, the hearing aid technology has continued to improve with respect to signal processing strategies, comfort, and aesthetics. However, there are certain limitations with respect to understanding speech in background noise.[6] With severe-to-profound hearing loss, hearing aids fail to provide complete auditory access, thus affecting the audibility and intelligibility of speech. Some children with appropriately fitted amplification devices fail to make expected progress with respect to listening and speech language milestones. In such a situation, a cochlear implant must be considered as an option as early as possible.[7]

Cochlear Implants

A cochlear implant is an electronic device that helps an individual with severe-to-profound hearing loss to hear sounds occurring in the environment.[8] It consists of an external component and surgically placed internal component **(Fig. 3)**. The external component consists of a microphone, sound processor, battery, and transmitter. The microphone receives the sounds from the environment and sends it to the processor, where it is digitally analyzed, separated into different frequency bands, and compressed into an electrical signal. The signal is then sent through the skin to the internal components via the transmitter. The surgically placed internal component consists of a receiver-stimulator, which accepts the signal from the transmitter. The internal

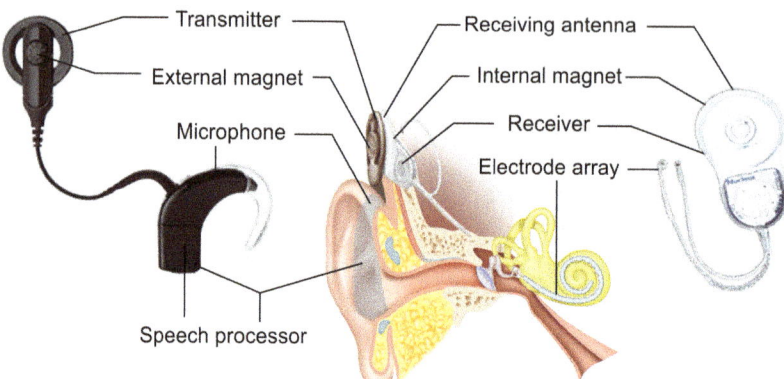

Fig. 3: Parts of cochlear implant.

receiver then delivers the signal to the electrode array which is inserted in the cochlea. The specific electrode will stimulate the auditory nerve through electric pulses. The internal and external components are connected to each other by a magnet which is attached to the transmitter and receiver-stimulator as well, thus allowing the signals to get conveyed across the skin. This basic working and parts of the cochlear implant are quite the same with different brands. However, they differ in terms of the external component designs, electrode arrays, and signal-processing strategies.

The cochlear implant is different from a hearing aid, as it is not an amplification device. It actually bypasses the damaged cochlea and directly stimulates the auditory nerve, thus helping the individual to hear sounds. Cochlear implants are indicated for children as young as 12 months of age who have bilateral severe–profound hearing loss and fail to show expected progress with the hearing aids.[3] Ching et al.[8] reported that young children who receive cochlear implants by 2 years of age have good outcomes, thus highlighting the importance of critical period of development. Cochlear implant candidacy is a joint process requiring teamwork from different professionals, i.e., cochlear implant surgeon, audiologist, radiologist, pediatrician, speech language therapist/special educator, and medical social worker. Cochlear implantation can be done bilaterally or unilaterally, along with a hearing aid in the other ear **(Fig. 4)**.

One major obstacle for cochlear implant decision-making in India is the cost of the implant. Majority of the parents are from low socioeconomic strata, thus self-funding for procuring cochlear implants is very difficult and most often families opt for unilateral implantation. The social worker has a crucial role in helping these families seek funding through non-governmental organizations or educating them regarding Central and State Government schemes where the cost of the implant surgery and further rehabilitation is provided completely free at no cost. The cost of maintenance and upgradation of the device has to be borne by the family. It is necessary to counsel the family regarding these aspects well in advance.

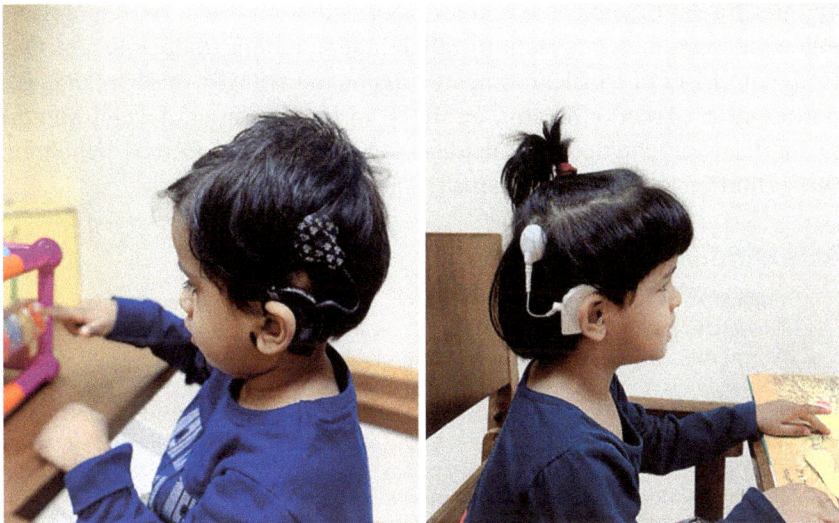

Fig. 4: Children fitted with unilateral cochlear implant.

AURAL HABILITATION

Aural habilitation involves teaching the child the skill to "learn to listen" with the hearing devices. As soon as the child is fitted with hearing devices, the audiologist refers the family to early intervention services where the speech language pathologist/speech therapist/teacher for the deaf/aural habilitationist works with the child and the family to help them communicate. One of the early decisions to be taken by the family for their child is regarding the communication mode, i.e., whether their child will use spoken language or sign language or a combination of both. With the advent of digital hearing aids and cochlear implants, majority of the parents expect their child to use spoken language to communicate. Thus, the primary goal of training is to develop spoken form of language through listening and acquire age-appropriate communication skills that are necessary for integration into mainstream schools and the hearing community. As each and every child is unique and has different learning styles, the communication outcomes will vary. There are several factors which will influence these outcomes, like the age of the child, involvement and motivation level of the parents, educational status of the parents (especially the mother), knowledge and skills of the professionals, availability of therapy services, regular follow-up, and travel time taken from families' hometown to the intervention center. Taking these aspects into consideration, the families need to be counseled appropriately regarding setting realistic expectations from their child. As habilitation professionals, our role is to guide and coach the parents of children with hearing loss, empower them, and help them identify the goals and aspirations for their child.

At the KEM Hospital, Pune, we started a cochlear implant center in 2006 with the objective of early identification of hearing loss and providing appropriate intervention services. The entire preimplant candidacy evaluation and postimplant management in terms of switch-on of the hearing device, follow-up mappings, and auditory rehabilitation is done under one roof. Our team comprises of cochlear implant surgeon, audiologist, speech language pathologist, special educator, auditory verbal therapist, developmental pediatrician, psychologist, and medical social worker. The focus is on helping these children to be a part of mainstream education and society.

REFERENCES

1. English K. Informing parents of their child's hearing loss: "Breaking Bad News" Guidelines for Audiologists. Audiology Today. 2004:16:10-2.
2. Northern J, Downs M. Hearing in Children, 4th edition. Baltimore: Williams and Wilkins; 1991.
3. Joint Committee on Infant Hearing. Year. Position Statement: Principles and Guidelines for Early Hearing Detection and Intervention Programs. J Early Hear Detect Interv. 2019;4;1-44.
4. Bagatto M, Moodie S, Brown C, Malandrino A, Richert F, Clench D, et al. Prescribing and verifying hearing aids applying the American Academy of Audiology Pediatric Amplification Guideline: Protocols and outcomes from the Ontario Infant Hearing Program. J Am Acad Audiol. 2016:27(3):188-203.
5. Lesica NA. Hearing aids: limitations and opportunities. Hear J. 2018:71(5):43-6.
6. Gifford RH. Who is a cochlear implant candidate? Hear J. 2011;64(6):18-22.
7. National Institute on Deafness and Other Communication Disorders (NIDCD) Fact Sheet: Cochlear Implants. February 2016.
8. Ching TYC, Dillon H, Day J, Crowe K, Close L, Chrisholm K, et al. Early language outcomes of children with cochlear implants: Interim findings of the NAL study on longitudinal outcomes of children with hearing impairment. Cochlear Implants Int. 2009;10(Suppl 1):28-32.

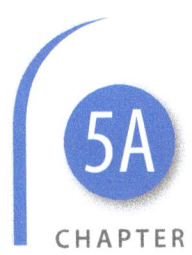

5A CHAPTER

Visual Impairment

Aditi Patwardhan

INTRODUCTION

Of all the five senses, vision is the most important sense which provides information to the brain. Only vision can perceive size, shape, color, distance, and spatial location in one glance. All the other senses put together cannot provide an equal amount of information to the brain. Retinopathy of prematurity (ROP) is the main ophthalmological problem in preterm infants. Other problems are refractive errors, strabismus, amblyopia, and cortical blindness.

Retinopathy of prematurity is a retinal vasoproliferative disease, which is seen exclusively in preterm infants.

EPIDEMIOLOGY: RETINOPATHY OF PREMATURITY

There are three distinct periods known as ROP "epidemics."

First ROP epidemic: It was seen in the 1940s and early 1950s, where larger and more mature infants showed blindness due to ROP. It was related to unrestricted oxygen administration with no means of monitoring its use.

Second ROP epidemic: It was seen in late 1960s and 1970s, when monitoring of oxygen saturation was developed with well-developed neonatal units where less mature infants, in particular those <1,000 g, showed blindness, due to ROP despite the improvements in technology and knowledge.

Third ROP epidemic: It was seen from 1990 onwards. Presently, India and other middle-income countries are facing the third epidemic of ROP. It is a combination of first and second epidemics, in which mature as well as immature preterm babies were affected. With varying levels of care in the community, some larger institutes provide the highest level of care, where only extremely premature infants develop ROP. Whereas in smaller towns and rural areas, where neonatal care units are proliferating rapidly, even larger and more mature infants suffer from the disease.[1,2]

PREVALENCE OF RETINOPATHY OF PREMATURITY IN INDIA

It is projected that approximately 18,000 infants will go blind every year in India due to ROP. India needs to gear up to face the challenge of the third epidemic and prevent ROP-related blindness by expanding the screening and treatment programs.

RISK FACTORS FOR RETINOPATHY OF PREMATURITY

Prematurity: Gestational age and birth weight are the two strongest known risk factors for development of ROP.[3,4]

Other risk factors include:
- Low Apgar score
- Respiratory distress syndrome (RDS) requiring surfactant and oxygen
- Prolonged mechanical ventilation
- Intraventricular hemorrhage (Grade III, IV)
- Sepsis
- Blood transfusion/exchange transfusion
- Patent ductus arteriosus needing closure

PATHOPHYSIOLOGY OF RETINOPATHY OF PREMATURITY

Retinopathy of prematurity is a two-phase disease.

Phase I (Vasoconstrictive Phase)

Phase I is characterized by delayed physiologic retinal vascular development and vasoattenuation. This phase occurs during exposure to high oxygen levels which cause suppression of the normal anterior-ward vascularization of the retina, and there is downregulation of vascular endothelial growth factor (VEGF).

Phase II (Vasoproliferative Phase)

Phase II is seen when phase I-induced hypoxia releases factors to stimulate new blood vessel growth. There is a sudden surge in VEGF levels. It causes dilatation and tortuosity of the existing larger vessels with neovascularization and proliferation of new vessels into the vitreous. VEGF and insulin-like growth factor-I (IGF-I) play a key role in pathogenesis of ROP.

Vascular endothelial growth factor is an important oxygen-regulated factor. A critical non-oxygen-regulated growth factor is IGF-I. IGF-I is essential for growth of the retinal vasculature. Low serum levels of IGF-I during the first weeks/months of life have been found to correlate with severity of ROP.

CLASSIFICATION OF RETINOPATHY OF PREMATURITY

The International Classification of Retinopathy of Prematurity (ICROP) categorizes ROP into stages (0–5), location of the disease in (zone 1–3), extent of the disease based on clock hours (1–12), and the presence of plus disease.

With better retinal imaging techniques, this classification was modified in 2005,[5] which introduced aggressive posterior retinopathy of prematurity (APROP), and pre-plus disease.

DISEASE LOCATION INTO ZONES

The three zones of ROP are centered on the optic disk **(Fig. 1)**.
1. Zone I is the small circle of retina around the optic disk. The radius of the circle is twice the distance from the macula to the center of the optic disk.
2. Zone II is the ring-shaped section of the retina surrounding zone I, which extends to the ora serrata on the nasal side.
3. Zone III is a crescent-shaped area of temporal retina.

DISEASE STAGES

Severity of the disease is determined by staging. More than one stage may be present in the same eye.
- *Stage 1 demarcation line:* A demarcation line is a thin, flat line seen between the vascular and avascular retina **(Fig. 2)**.
- *Stage 2 ridge:* A ridge **(Fig. 3)** is a three-dimensional structure which arises from the demarcation line and extends above the retina. Small tufts of new vessels also called as "popcorn" vessels **(Fig. 4)** may be seen posterior to the ridge.
- *Stage 3 extraretinal fibrovascular proliferation:* Extraretinal fibrovascular proliferation or neovascularization extends into the vitreous from the ridge **(Fig. 5)**. It may be continuous or noncontinuous and is posterior to the ridge.
- *Stage 4 subtotal or partial retinal detachment:* It is divided into two stages—extrafoveal or fovea sparing **(Fig. 6)** and fovea involving
- *Stage 5:* Total retinal detachment **(Fig. 7)**

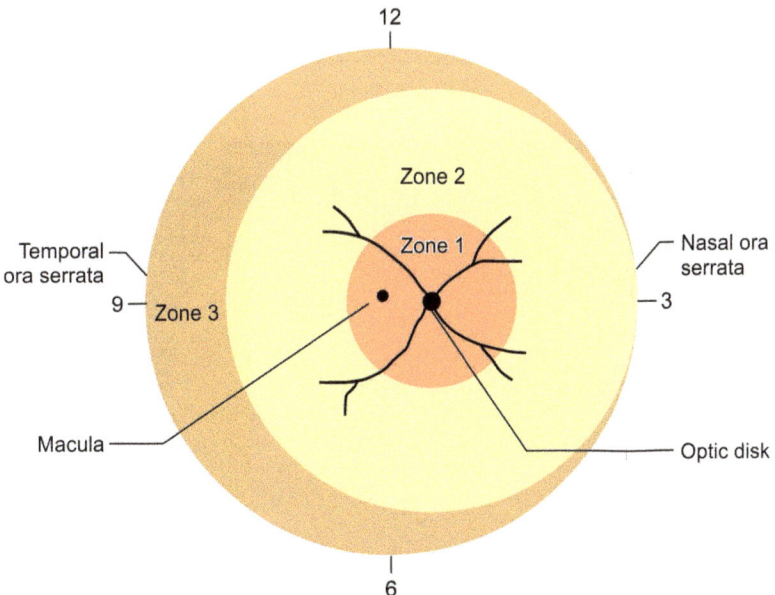

Fig. 1: Zones of retinopathy of prematurity (ROP).

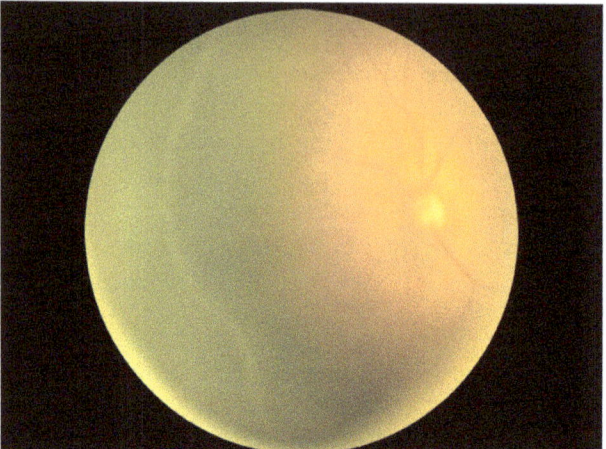

Fig. 2: Demarcation line.

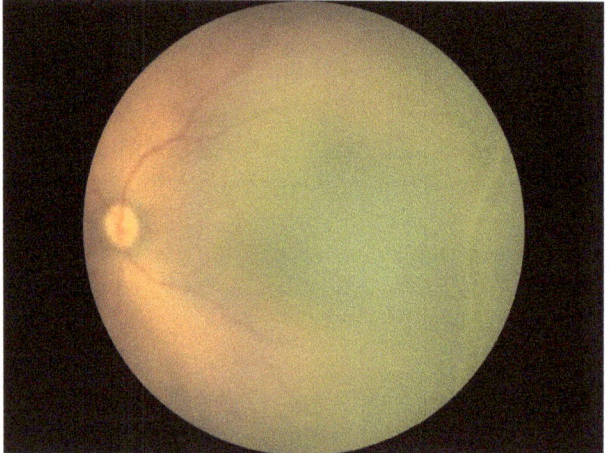

Fig. 3: Ridge.

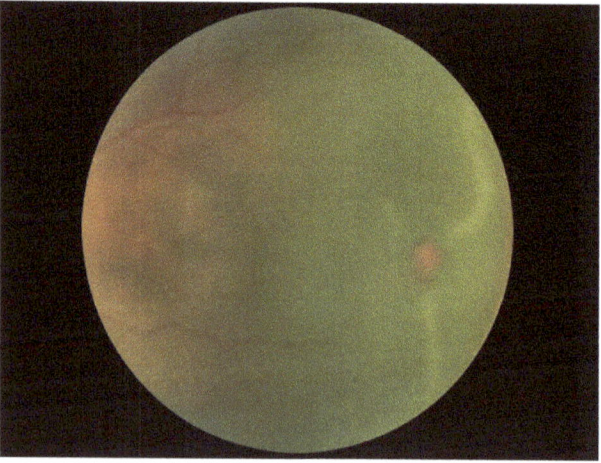

Fig. 4: Ridge with popcorn vessels.

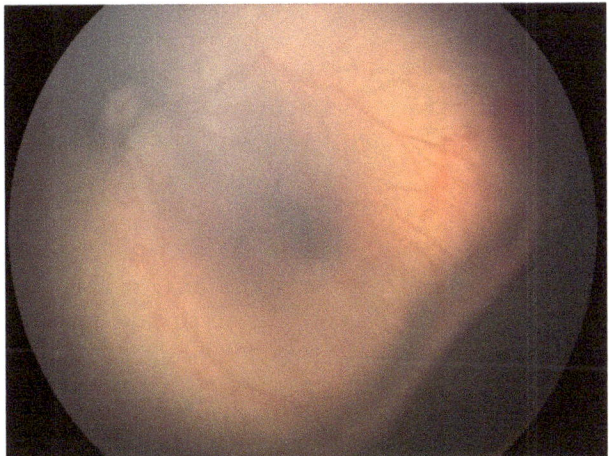

Fig. 5: New vessels growing toward vitreous.

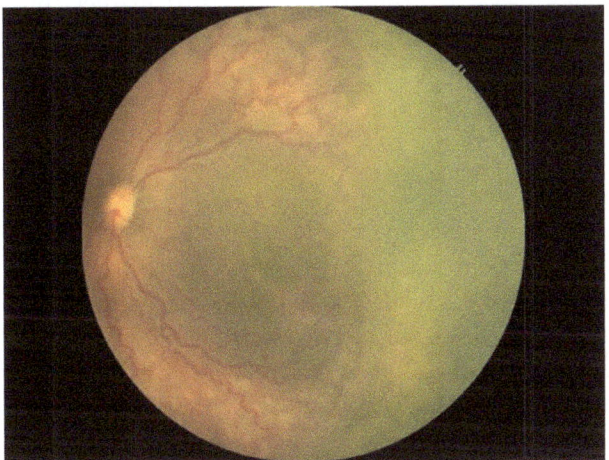

Fig. 6: Fovea sparing partial retinal detachment.

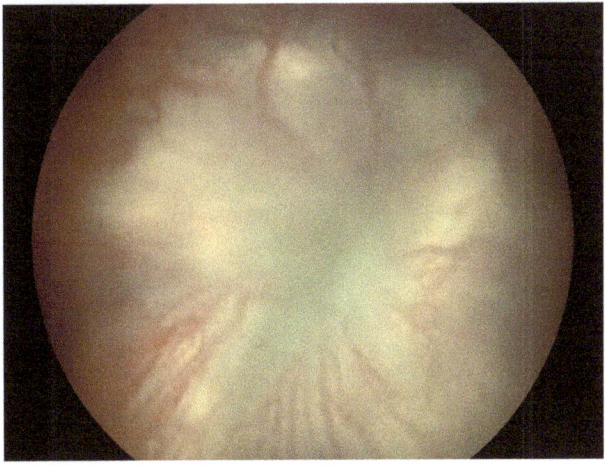

Fig. 7: Total retinal detachment.

EXTENT OF RETINOPATHY

The extent of the ROP is documented by the number of clock hours involved from 1 to 12 with each clock hour at 30°.

Following signs indicate that ROP is active.

Plus Disease

Plus disease is defined as arterial tortuosity and venous dilation in the posterior pole blood vessels **(Fig. 8)**. Two quadrants of the retina must be involved for the changes to be characterized as plus disease. It is an indicator of severity of the disease and is the most critical finding in identifying ROP requiring treatment.

Aggressive Posterior Retinopathy of Prematurity

Aggressive posterior retinopathy of prematurity is characterized by severe plus disease, flat neovascularization in zone 1 or posterior zone 2, intraretinal shunting, hemorrhages, and a rapid progression to retinal detachment[5] **(Fig. 9)**.

Aggressive posterior retinopathy of prematurity has poor prognosis despite early treatment and is generally seen in preterm infants with gestational age (GA) <28 weeks and birth weight <1,000 g.

SCREENING FOR RETINOPATHY OF PREMATURITY

Early detection and timely intervention to reduce the burden of blindness make screening an important aspect of ROP. There is a lack of gold standard for screening criteria as the disease requires detailed understanding of the infants at risk and timely identification, which differs in different parts of world.

The screening guidelines published by Rashtriya Bal Swasthya Karyakram, Ministry of Health and Family Welfare, Government of India, June 2017, are as follows:[6]

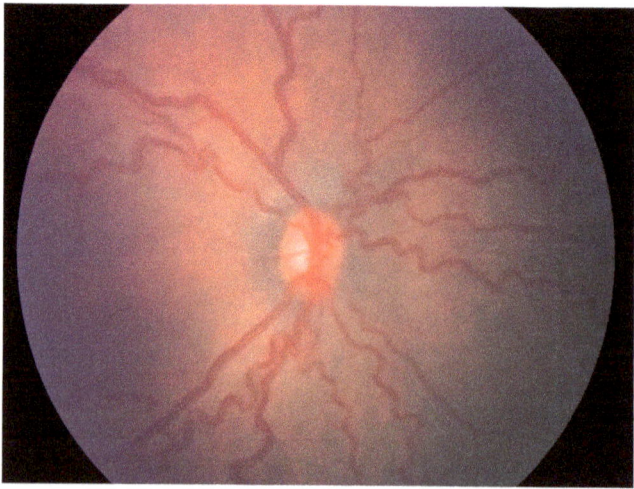

Fig. 8: Arterial tortuosity and venous dilation in all quadrants.

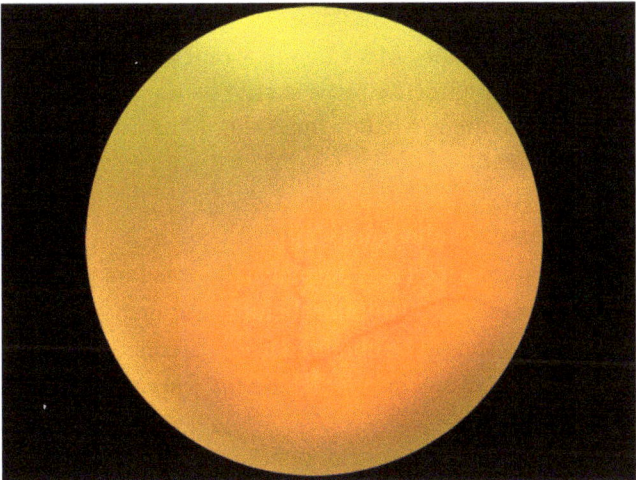

Fig. 9: Flat neovascularization is seen in superior quadrant.

- Infants with any of the following factors are screened:
  - Birth weight <2,000 g
  - Gestational age <34 weeks
  - Gestational age between 34 and 36 weeks but with risk factors such as: (1) cardiorespiratory support, (2) prolonged oxygen therapy, (3) RDS, (4) chronic lung disease, (5) fetal hemorrhage, (6) blood transfusion, (7) neonatal sepsis, (8) exchange transfusion, (9) intraventricular hemorrhage, (10) apneas, and (11) poor postnatal weight gain
  - Infants with an unstable clinical course who are at high-risk (as determined by the neonatologist or pediatrician)

Timing to Screen[6]
- Should receive first screening at 4 weeks after birth
- Infants with gestation <28 weeks or weight <1,200 g should be first screened at 2–3 weeks after delivery.

Duration and Frequency of Screening
The screening examinations will continue at least every 2 weeks until:
- Vascularization of the retina reaches normal completion
- Until ROP regresses
- Until ROP requiring treatment develops

Pupillary Dilatation
Pupillary dilatation is required for meticulous examination of retina. Most commonly used dilating drops are a combination of phenylephrine (5%) and tropicamide (0.8%)—this should be diluted 1:1 with pharmaceutically available methyl cellulose eye drops, so that the final drops have 2.5% phenylephrine and 0.4% tropicamide.

Place to Screen

Neonates should be examined in the neonatal unit itself under supervision of the attending neonatologist. The place should be warm and clean. If babies are being screened in the eye clinic, there should be arrangement for basic resuscitation equipment.

The examination procedure is as follows:[6]
- Baby should be well clothed and wrapped.
- Baby should receive a feed and burped an hour before screening.
- Pupils should be dilated 30 minutes before examination.
- Informed consent should be obtained from parents.
- Topical anesthetic drops, proparacaine 0.5% should be applied at the conjunctival sac.
- A sterile wire lid speculum is put for opening of the eye after putting topical anesthesia and scleral indenter is used for eye rotation.
- The use of oral sucrose may be considered to help with analgesia.
- Screening should be done by an ophthalmologist trained in ROP screening.

Screening Documentation

Screening documentation should include:
- The zone of vascularization
- The stage of ROP
- The extent of ROP (in clock hours)
- The presence of plus or pre-plus disease
- The presence of APROP
- Whether treatment is indicated, or when follow-up is planned

Telescreening

Telescreening uses a wide-field digital camera for screening.

It is coming up as an important tool for ROP screening. Images can be captured by non-ophthalmologists like the neonatal nurses or technicians after training. This is important in areas that do not have ready access to pediatric ophthalmologists,[7] as captured images can be transferred electronically. As the images are stored and can be retrieved, it is also advantageous from a medicolegal perspective. The parents' compliance for treatment is better when we show the images to them. Parents then get more convinced for treatment and frequent follow-ups.

The limitation of telescreening is issues with image quality which is an important factor for effective and reliable ROP screening. The high cost of a wide-field imaging camera is a limiting factor for its widespread use.

TREATMENT

Timely treatment for ROP is critical to prevent severe vision impairment. The treatment is carried out to remove the stimulus for growth of new blood vessels

TABLE 1: Follow-up and treatment protocol according to ETROP (early treatment for retinopathy of prematurity) guidelines.

		Stage of ROP	Treatment recommended
ZONE I	No plus	Stage 1	Follow-up (1 week)
		Stage 2	Follow-up (1 week)
		Stage 3	Treat
	Plus	Stage 1	Treat
		Stage 2	Treat
		Stage 3	Treat
ZONE II	No plus	Stage 1	Follow-up (1–2 weeks)
		Stage 2	Follow-up (1–2 weeks)
		Stage 3	Follow-up (1–2 weeks)
	Plus	Stage 1	Follow-up (1–2 weeks)
		Stage 2	Follow-up (1–2 weeks)
		Stage 3	Treat

(ROP: retinopathy of prematurity)

by burning the peripheral avascular retina, which decreases the secretion of VEGF; resulting in regression of established ROP. Retinal ablation can be achieved by laser therapy. Laser allows more precision of treatment.

ETROP GUIDELINES FOR RETINOPATHY OF PREMATURITY LASER[8]

Not all ROP babies need treatment. ROP babies who need treatment are described in **Table 1**.

LASER TREATMENT

Laser is done using an indirect laser ophthalmoscope by an ophthalmologist trained in ROP laser, under topical anesthesia after pupillary dilatation. Treatment[9] is done either in the neonatal intensive care unit (NICU) or in an operating room equipped with suction apparatus and intubation equipment in the rare event of apnea or cardiac arrest. A neonatologist or anesthesiologist must be available on call. During the laser procedure, a pulse oximeter should monitor the baby. The entire avascular retina up to the ora serrata should be ablated with near confluent burns (0.5–1 burn width apart) up to the ridge **(Figs. 10 and 11)**.

In a single session, 3,000–4,000 spots may be required to ablate an avascular retina. In severe forms of the disease, posterior laser is given posterior to the ridge which helps in rapid and complete regression of disease.

Post laser, topical antibiotics and steroids are prescribed three times a day for 7 days to reduce any inflammation. Usually post-laser weekly reviews are recommended till complete ROP regression is seen. Few cases may require additional laser to skip areas. The most common side effects of laser treatment are myopia and peripheral restriction of vision.

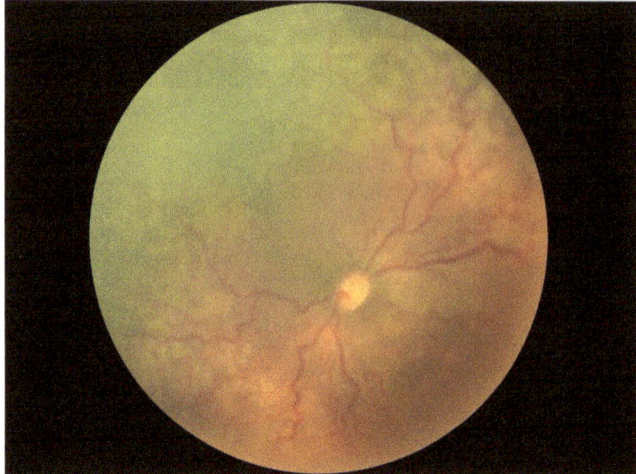

Fig. 10: Fresh, confluent laser marks.

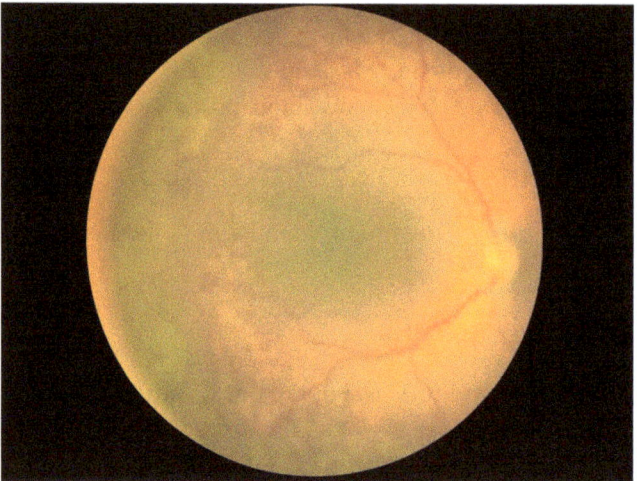

Fig. 11: Laser marks given posterior to ridge.

Antivascular Endothelial Growth Factor Drugs

Antivascular endothelial growth factor drugs act by blocking the action of VEGF which is a potent proangiogenic factor, thus reducing vascular activity. Anti-VEGF drugs are helpful as they act by rapidly regressing ROP. Other advantages are growth of retinal vasculature beyond the demarcation line, lesser degree of myopia and peripheral visual field loss, and avoidance of sedation and intubation required for laser.

However, it is still not the first choice of treatment as these drugs are short-acting and late recurrences can be seen. There are controversies regarding choice of anti-VEGF agent, dosing, systemic absorption, and safety.

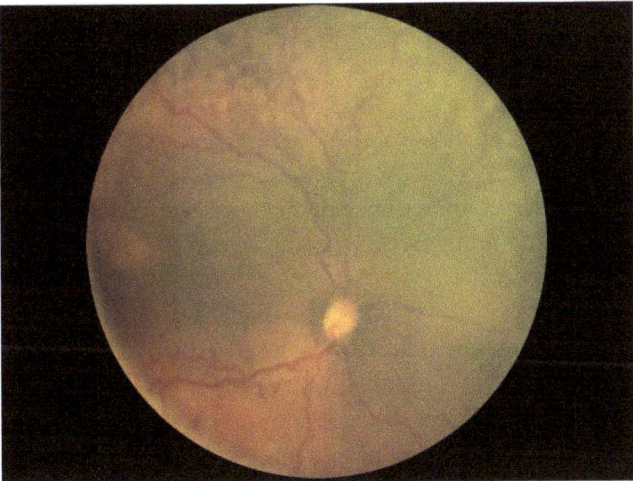

Fig. 12: Persisting plus disease after adequate laser.

At present, use of anti-VEGF drugs is restricted in the following situations:
- ROP progresses despite laser treatment **(Fig. 12)**
- When laser is not possible due to hazy media
- As a preoperative measure in retinal detachment with high vascularity, to reduce intraoperative bleeding

Most commonly used drugs are bevacizumab (avastin) and ranibizumab (accentrix).

The BEAT-ROP (Bevacizumab Eliminates the Angiogenic Threat of ROP) study[10] is the only randomized trial done comparing anti-VEGF versus conventional laser. It suggested the superiority of anti-VEGF treatment over conventional laser therapy for stage 3+ ROP in zone I, but not for zone II disease. This trial was too small to assess safety of bevacizumab in terms of local or systemic toxicity.

RAINBOW (Ranibizumab versus laser therapy for the treatment of very low birth weight infants with retinopathy of prematurity) study[11] has suggested that, ranibizumab 0.2 mg might be superior to laser therapy, with fewer unfavorable ocular outcomes than laser therapy and with an acceptable 24-week safety profile.

SURGICAL MANAGEMENT OF RETINOPATHY OF PREMATURITY

Surgical management of ROP is reserved only for advanced stages of ROP (stages 4 and 5) as the results are not encouraging.

Vitreoretinal surgery is associated with poor visual outcomes. Anatomical and visual successes are better for stage 4A ROP than stages 4B or 5 ROP.[12] Commonly used surgical techniques include microincision vitrectomy surgery (MIVS) with wide angle viewing systems for stage 4 and 5 ROP. Lens-sparing vitrectomy is preferred for stage 4A ROP. Primary scleral buckling can be also used for stage 4A ROP.[12]

OTHER CAUSES OF VISUAL IMPAIRMENT

Refractive Errors

The incidence of refractive errors is high even without ROP in preterm infants. Most of these infants are hyperopic, however, preterm infants with ROP have myopia. All infants who are premature should be referred for dilated eye examination to rule out refractive errors. Timely treatment of refractive errors provides significant improvement in visual acuity.

Strabismus

Children, who are very premature, are at a higher risk of strabismus compared to children born at term. A study by VanderVeen et al.[13] has shown that 14% of preterm infants had strabismus at 2 years and 80% of these have esotropia. This is particularly so in infants born before 26 weeks gestation or in infants with severe intrauterine growth restriction.

Infants born at a gestation <32 weeks should be advised long-term ophthalmologic follow-up. Parents should be counseled regarding the importance of this follow-up. All these infants should be screened at 1 year, in the third year (preferably around 30 months), and just before school entry for visual acuity.

Amblyopia

It is also known as "lazy eye syndrome," where vision in one eye is reduced due to abnormal visual development in childhood. Amblyopia in preterm infants is caused by undiagnosed or late diagnosis of refractive errors or strabismus. A long-term follow-up study from Saudi Arabia showed a high incidence of myopia and astigmatism in children who had ROP.[14]

Cortical Blindness

An infant's early development depends on vision, since all other systems require a visual feedback for practice and refinement. Visual information cannot be provided to the infant if either the brain or the eyes are dysfunctional. The two systems are closely interconnected, hence, visual stimulation has to start early. Incorporation of other senses such as hearing, touch, and smell into the visual experiences helps the child make better sense of visual images. Some motor milestones which are usually visually guided may be late in these children and may need special training. The parents must arrange a room that is bright and full of color. Some decorative colorful items and some noise-making toys may be kept in the room, which can be banged, kicked, or dropped. The blind child should not be overprotected, but treated like a normal child.

REFERENCES

1. Hungi B, Vinekar A, Datti N, Kariyappa P, Braganza S, Chinnaiah S, et al. Retinopathy of prematurity in a rural neonatal intensive care unit in South India: a prospective study. Indian J Pediatr. 2012;79(7):911-15.

2. Vinekar A, Jayadev C, Mangalesh S, Shetty B, Vidyasagar D. Role of tele-medicine in retinopathy of prematurity screening in rural outreach centers in India: a report of 20,214 imaging sessions in the KIDROP program. Semin Fetal Neonatal Med. 2015;20(5):335-45.
3. Shah VA, Yeo CL, Ling YL. Incidence, risk factors of retinopathy of prematurity among very low birth weight infants in Singapore. Ann Acad Med Singapore. 2005;34(2):169-78.
4. Liu PM, Fang PC, Huang CB, Kou HK, Chung MY, Yang YH, et al. Risk factors of retinopathy of prematurity in premature infants weighing less than 1600 g. Am J Perinatol. 2005;22(2):115-20.
5. International Committee for the Classification of Retinopathy of Prematurity. The International Classification of Retinopathy of Prematurity revisited. Arch Ophthalmol. 2005;123(7):991-9.
6. Government of India. Revised_ROP_Guidelines-Web_Optimized Guidelines for universal eye screening in newborns including Retinopathy of prematurity. [online] Available from: https://nhm.gov.in/images/pdf/programmes/RBSK/Resource_Documents/Revised_ROP_Guidelines-Web_Optimized.pdf. [Last accessed January, 2021].
7. Kandasamy Y, Smith R, Wright I, Hartley L. Use of digital retinal imaging in screening for retinopathy of prematurity. J Paediatr Child Health. 2013;49(1):E1-5.
8. Early Treatment of Prematurity Cooperative Group. Revised indications for treatment of retinopathy of prematurity: results of early treatment of retinopathy of prematurity randomized trial. Arch Ophalmol. 2003;121(12):1684-94.
9. Jalali S, Azad R, Trehan HS, Dogra MR, Gopal L, Narendran V. Technical aspects of laser treatment for acute retinopathy of prematurity under topical anesthesia. Ophthalmology Practice. 2010;58(6):509-15.
10. Mintz-Hittner HA, Kennedy KA, Chuang AZ; BEAT-ROP Cooperative Group. Efficacy of intravitreal bevacizumab for stage 3+ retinopathy of prematurity. N Engl J Med. 2011;364(7):603-15.
11. Stahl A, Lepore D, Fielder A, Fleck B, Reynolds JD, Chiang MF, et al. Ranibizumab versus laser therapy for the treatment of very low birthweight infants with retinopathy of prematurity (RAINBOW): an open-label randomised controlled trial. Lancet. 2019;394(10208):1551-9.
12. Shah PK, Narendran V, Kalpana N, Tawansy KA. Anatomical and visual outcome of stages 4 and 5 retinopathy of prematurity. Eye. 2009;23(1):176-80.
13. VanderVeen DK, Allred EN, Wallace DK, Leviton A, Strabismus at age 2 years in children born before 28 weeks' gestation: Antecedents and correlates J Child Neurol. 2016;31(4):451-60.
14. Bin-Khathlan AA, Al-Ballaa FN, AlYahya AK. Ophthalmic short- and long-terms for premature infants: results of an extended program in Saudi Arabia. Saudi J Ophthalmol. 2014;28(4):268-73.

CHAPTER 5B

Retinopathy of Prematurity in a Tertiary Care Center: Incidence, Risk Factors, and Follow-up*

Sudha Chaudhari

A large prospectives study to find out the incidence of retinopathy of prematurity (ROP) in a tertiary care center was done at the KEM Hospital, Pune, by Chaudhari et al.[1] The study attempted to identify the risk factors which predispose to ROP in a large population of NICU graduates and also the long-term outcome of those treated with laser therapy.

Neonates weighing <1,500 g and/or with a gestation <32 weeks admitted to the neonatal intensive care unit (NICU) were screened for ROP between the years 2000 and 2006. Neonates with birth weight >1,500 g or gestational age >32 weeks were screened only if they had an unstable course in the NICU with risk factors such as ventilation, respiratory distress syndrome (RDS) with use of surfactant, septicemia, intraventricular hemorrhage, hyperbilirubinemia, exchange transfusion, apnea, and use of blood products. The screening was done by the same ophthalmologist in all neonates and retinopathy was graded.

Infants with normal vascularization up to periphery were not examined again. Those with ROP were examined every week till regression had occurred or threshold for laser treatment had reached. Stage 3 ROP with plus disease with 5 contiguous clock hours or a total of 8 noncontiguous clock hours in zones 1 and 2 was considered for treatment. All children who received laser treatment were followed up very regularly. At the age of 3 years, they were recalled for a detailed ophthalmic examination.

550 infants were screened for ROP during this period. Their mean birth weight was 1306 ± 267 g and their mean gestation was 31.4 ± 2.2. The overall incidence of ROP was 22.3%. The incidence of ROP according to gestational age is shown in **Figure 1**. The incidence of ROP in 58 ELBW infants was 36.2% and 23.8% in 381 VLBW infants. No ROP was seen in infants weighing >2,000 g. **Table 1** shows the distribution of stages of ROP.

There was no predilection for sex. There was no difference in ROP between appropriate for gestational age (AGA) and small for gestational age (SGA) infants.

A univariate analysis was done taking each risk factor. Septicemia (0.003), apnea (0.0001), oxygen therapy (0.0001), ventilation, and use of blood products (p = 0.013) were found to be significant risk factors. When analyzed with a multiple regression, only apnea, septicemia, and oxygen therapy were found to be significant risk factors. Out of the 123 infants having ROP, laser therapy

---

*This is a summary of an article published in "Indian Pediatrics" by the author.

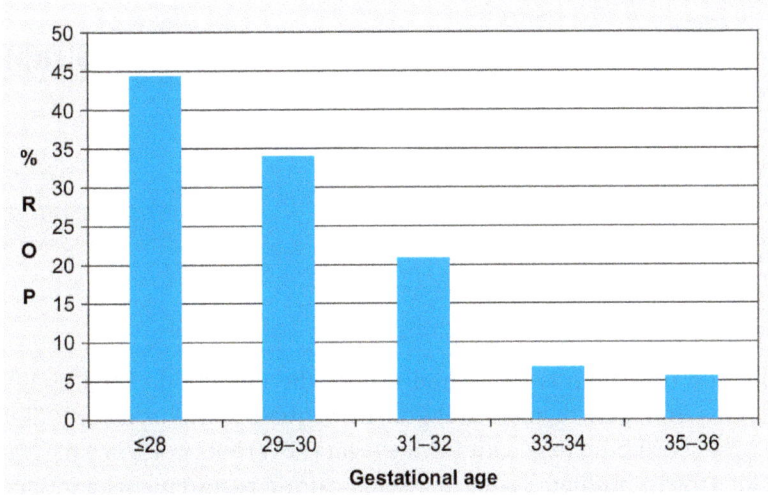

Fig. 1: Incidence of retinopathy of prematurity (ROP) according to gestational age.

TABLE 1: Frequency distribution of stages of retinopathy of prematurity (ROP).

Stages	Left eye n (%)	Right eye n (%)
I	46 (39.6)	49 (39.8)
II	40 (34.5)	43 (34.9)
III	23 (20.2)	23 (18.7)
IV	5 (4.4)	6 (4.9)
V	2 (1.7)	2 (1.6)
Total	116	123

was done in 41 (33.3%). All babies withstood the procedure without having any complications. Reddening of the conjunctiva disappeared in 2–3 days.

An effort was made to recall all children who had undergone laser therapy, at the age of 3 years. About 22 children (53.6%) had a complete ophthalmic check-up. Ten children had myopia and needed glasses and one had amblyopia, and 9 children had completely normal structural and visual outcome. Two children (9%) had poor outcome, 1 girl had retinal detachment in one eye and is blind in one eye. Another boy had retinal detachment in both eyes and is totally blind.

Since ROP is initially asymptomatic in the early stages, it is mandatory that carefully timed retinal examination of at-risk infants for ROP by a trained ophthalmologist be done, to minimize visual loss in these infants.

REFERENCE

1. Chaudhari S, Patwardhan V, Vaidya U, Kadam S, Kamat A. Retinopathy of prematurity in a tertiary care center: incidence, risk factors and outcome. Indian Pediatr. 2009;46(3):219-24.

CHAPTER 6A: Growth and Development

Sudha Chaudhari

INTRODUCTION

Evaluation of growth is very important in the follow-up of the high-risk newborns. Poor growth may result from inadequate nutrition, chronic illness, or psychosocial problems. Low birth weight (LBW) babies are at a particular risk for growth problems with increased caloric requirements and factors which impair intake. So it is crucial to ensure adequate and optimum intake and monitor growth parameters very closely.

The factors affecting growth in the LBW infants are as follows:
- *Increased caloric requirement*: Caloric requirements for the preterm infant are more, particularly during "catch-up" growth.
- *Increased losses*: Malabsorption may result from bowel resection done for necrotizing enterocolitis in the neonatal intensive care unit (NICU). Gastroesophageal reflux may cause chronic vomiting.
- *Decreased intake*: This may result from hypoxemia, oral motor dysfunction, or fatigue.
- *Intrinsic growth retardation*: Many LBW infants with intrauterine growth retardation (IUGR) do not achieve normal growth.

GROWTH EXPECTATIONS

When evaluating the growth and development of a preterm infant, it is essential to adjust the age for prematurity by the formula, chronologic age minus number of weeks born prematurely = corrected age, when one is using conventional growth charts. Head circumference, length, and weight should be measured and plotted every month.

GROWTH OUTCOME

Infants generally stabilize after the initial acute neonatal course. Then, they enter the phase of accelerated growth called the "catch-up" growth. This generally occurs in the first 2 years of life. Optimal nutrition is very important during this phase.

GROWTH PATTERNS

Low birth weight appropriate for gestational age (AGA) infants generally show catch-up growth during the first 2–3 years. Little catch-up growth occurs after

3 years of chronological age.[1] The head circumference is the first parameter to catch up, often plotting on higher centiles than weight and length. The rapid catch-up growth of the head must be distinguished from the pathological head growth of hydrocephalus. Calculating a length-to-head circumference ratio might help. A ratio of 1.42 or 1.48 is within normal limits, whereas a ratio 1.12 to 1.32 is abnormal.

The small for gestational age (SGA) LBW infants have less catch-up growth **(Fig. 1)**. They have less than normal weight and length at 3 years. Those who show some catch-up growth do so by 8–12 months corrected age. The head circumference is the first parameter to catch up. The "Pune Low Birth Weight

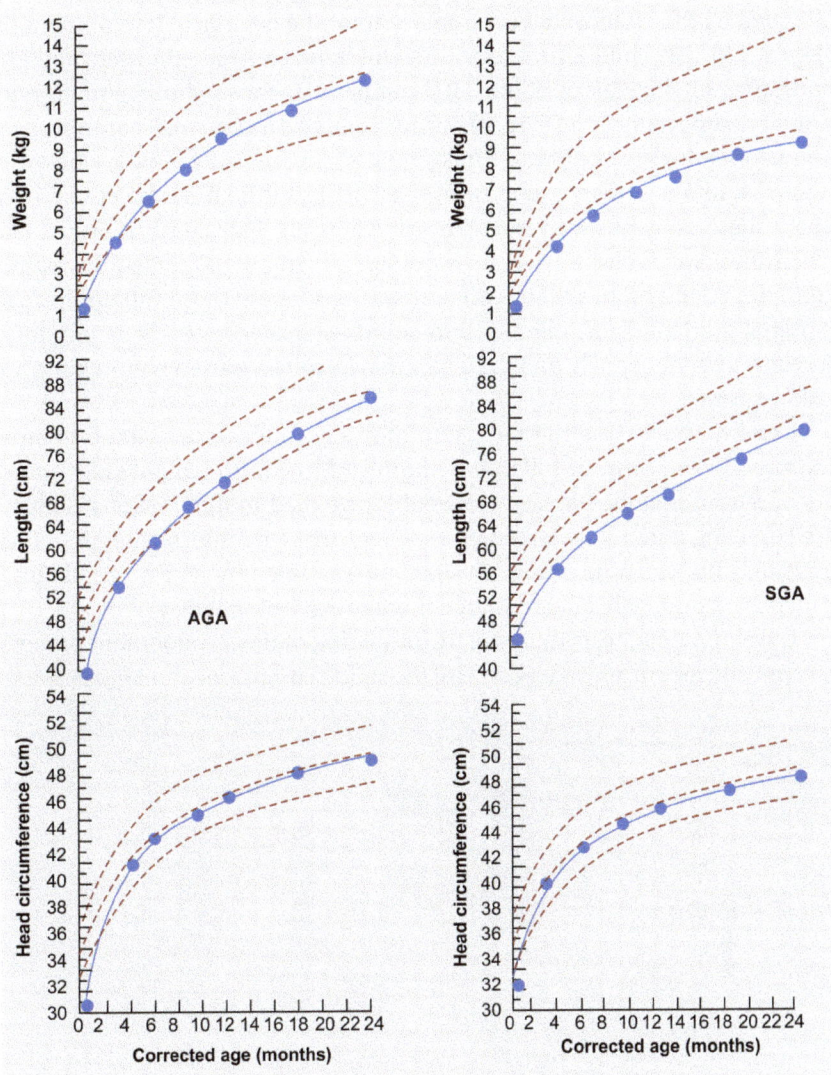

Fig. 1: Typical growth chart of low birth weight (LBW) appropriate for gestational age (AGA) and small for gestational age (SGA) infants.

Study" has shown that SGA LBW children were lighter, shorter, and had smaller head circumference compared to normal controls at 12 years.[2] Anthropometric measurements should be taken every month and plotted on "Intergrowth 21" charts till 52 weeks and subsequently on the World Health Organization (WHO) charts. This gives a correct perspective of the growth of the child.

NEURODEVELOPMENTAL ASSESSMENT

Development is a multiphasic and multifactorial phenomenon. It is influenced by two major factors—the biological risks and the environmental risks. In early infancy, it is the risk factors at birth that are important and later on it is the environment in which the child grows up. In an article entitled "Biology versus Environment,"[3] we have shown that parental education and type of school attended by the child were very important for the cognitive development of 12-year-old LBW children. Preterm SGA children of college-educated mothers had higher intelligence quotients (IQ) compared to those whose mothers had primary school education **(Fig. 2)**. Birth weight had a very small contribution. The neonatologist should not think that his responsibility is over when the high-risk infant is discharged from the NICU. But he must be concerned about the quality of survival as the survival itself. This concept originated when Sheridan published her paper in 1962, "Infants at risk for handicapping conditions." Sheridan's main concern was to identify these infants so that parental guidance and intervention could be started as early as possible. It is only after her epoch-making paper that hospitals started maintaining "at risk" registers.

Cerebral palsy was the most common neurodevelopmental outcome reported in the past, in follow-up studies of low birth weight (LBW) and very preterm infants. Babies who would have died in the previous century are surviving and a new generation of "high-risk" infants is emerging. It is extremely important to follow these infants, so that infants who need close supervision and early interventional therapy can be identified.

Developmental tests measure the unfolding of the development process and provide the current assessment of the child's competence and functioning.

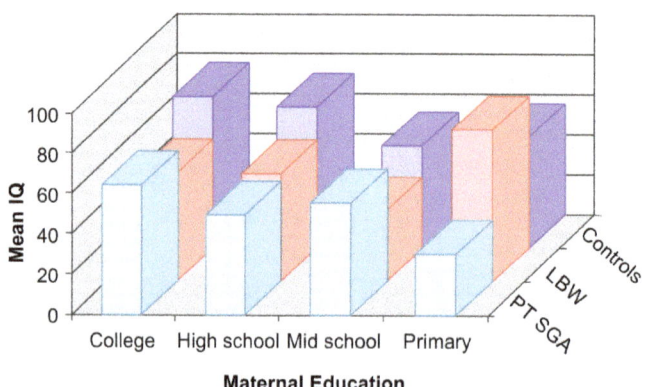

Fig. 2: Maternal education and intelligence quotient (IQ).

Hence, the assessments should be longitudinal and no conclusions should be drawn from a single examination. Just as you need a period of convalescence after recovering from any major illness, the high-risk infant's brain needs a little time to recover from the traumas in the NICU. So the first formal assessment should be done when the child is 3 months old. A developmental assessment should never be done when the child is hungry, sleepy, or ill. All assessments in infancy should be done using the corrected age in preterms.

AMIEL-TISON NEUROLOGICAL ASSESSMENT
Age (1–12 months) (Time approximately 10 minutes)

This test can be easily learnt by the neonatologists. Developmental tests such as the Developmental Assessment Scales for Indian Infants (DASII) can be used. But these tests are time-consuming, need a special kit and a sound-proof room and a well-trained psychologist. Hence, the need for a test of neurological evaluation, which can be easily learnt by neonatologists, was felt. Andre Thomas described one such test in 1949. This was studied extensively by Saint-Anne Dargassies in France and later presented in a tabulated form by Claudine Amiel-Tison.[4] By this method, the neurological condition of each child can be described objectively according to clearly defined standards, from a structured neurological examination.

Evaluation of muscle tone is a fundamental part of the study. A clear understanding of the evolution of tone is necessary to interpret this test. The upper limbs begin to relax and acquire skills before the lower limbs. In the axis, head control appears first, followed by the ability to sit, stand and finally walk by 12–18 months. Thus, from knowledge of the successive stages of maturation throughout the sequence, it is possible to identify abnormal clusters of response indicating deviant development.

The following data is noted before evaluating the tone (**Annexure I**):
- Examination of skull for sutures, size of anterior fontanelle and head circumference. The waxing and waning pattern of neuromotor development from 28 weeks to the end of the first year should be clearly understood. For example, from 28 to 40 weeks of gestation, the acquisition of muscle tone and motor function spreads from the lower extremities to the head (caudocephalic). After full term, the process is reversed, so that relaxation and motor control proceed downward for the next 12–18 months (cephalocaudal) (**Figs. 3 and 4**).
- Abnormal ocular signs such as hypertonia of levator palpebrae superioris, strabismus, and nystagmus
- Neurosensory development is assessed by noting visual pursuit by a red ball and hearing with a bell.
- Information is collected from the mother regarding convulsions during the preceding months and sleeping patterns.
- Arousal patterns, quality of cry, sucking, and swallowing behavior can be noted during the examination.

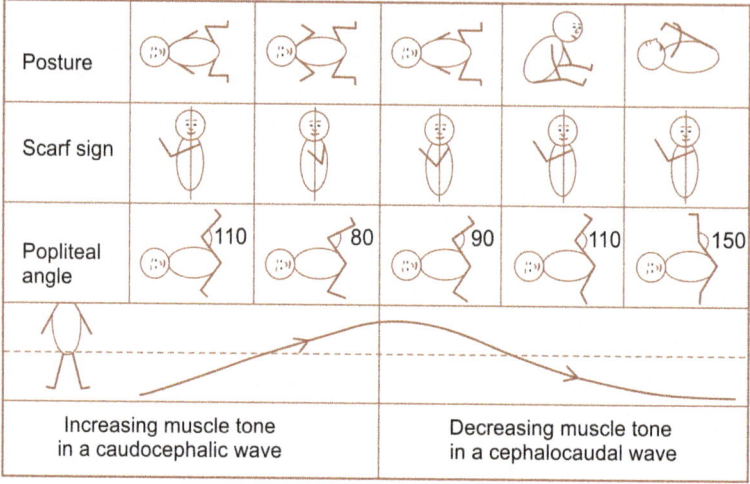

Fig. 3: Passive tone.

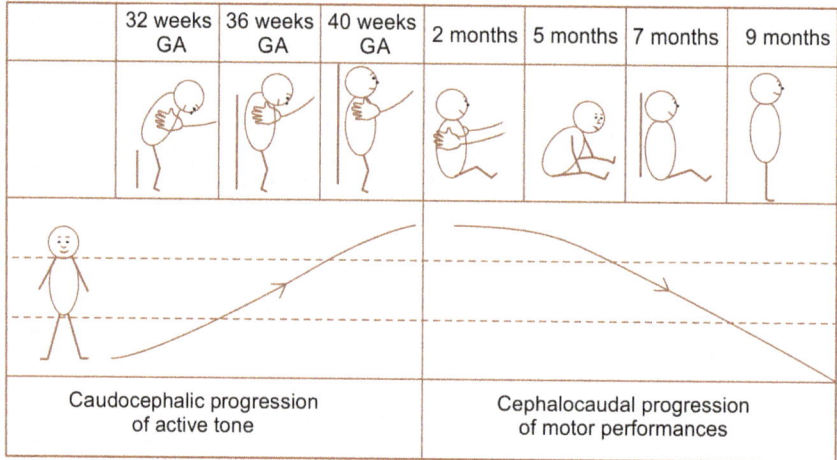

Fig. 4: Active tone.

- The evaluation of tone is based on the study of spontaneous posture, passive tone, and active tone.
- Axillary suspension should be done before assessing the tone. A hypotonic infant will slip through the hands, a spastic infant may spontaneously scissor **(Fig. 5)**.
- Spontaneous posture is studied by inspecting the child while he lies undisturbed **(Fig. 6)**.
- Passive tone is evaluated by applying certain maneuvers to an extremity. The resistance of the extremity to the maneuver is measured as an angle **(Fig. 7)**.
- The angles are the same as those used in Ballard's gestational age score such as the adductor angle, popliteal angle, and scarf sign.

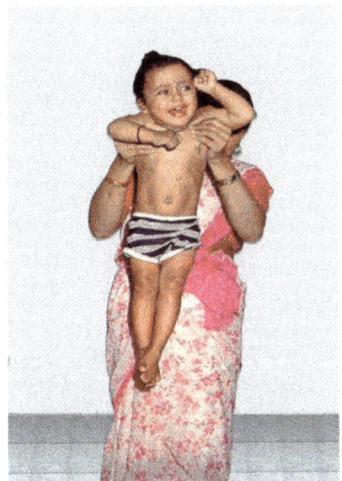

Fig. 5: Axillary suspension.

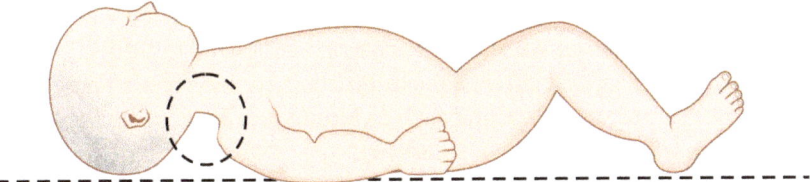

Fig. 6: Abnormal hypertonia of neck extensor muscles.

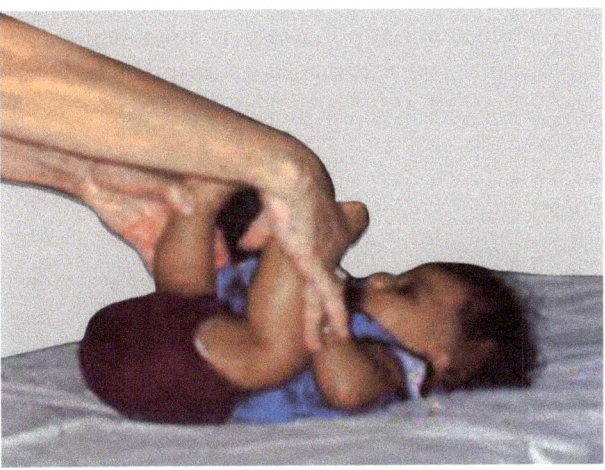

Fig. 7: Popliteal angle.

- Active tone is studied with the infant moving spontaneously in response to a given stimulus like pull to sit or pull to stand.

The infant should be awake, not crying, lying straight with the head in the midline while doing these maneuvers. All assessments are done using corrected or postconceptional age and not chronological age, thereby permitting the assessment of the preterm and the full-term infants by the same criteria.

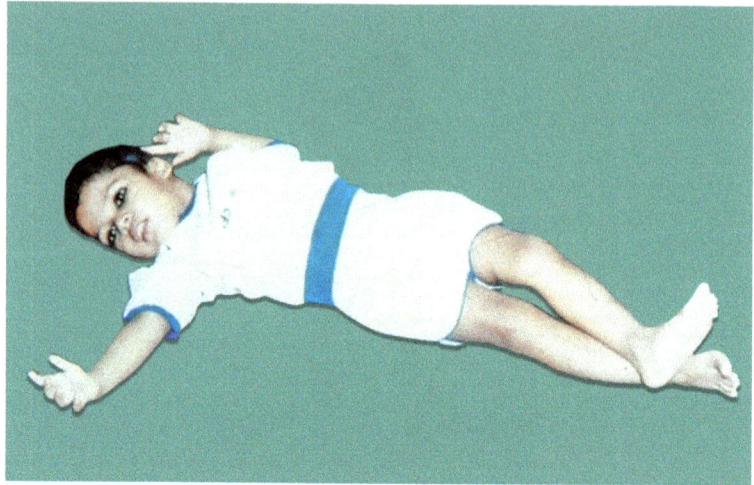

Fig. 8: Spontaneous asymmetrical tonic neck reflex (ATNR) in spastic cerebral palsy (CP).

Reflexes are also studied. Brisk tendon reflexes and clonus are noted. The persistence of primitive reflexes such as asymmetrical tonic neck reflex is especially looked for **(Fig. 8)**. Fisting and cortical thumb are also noted. The appearance of postural reactions such as lateral propping and parachute at the right age is also noted **(Figs. 9 and 10)**.

All this information put together makes it a complete neurological examination. With a little bit of practice, the entire examination can be completed in just 10 minutes. Although monthly evaluation is described by Amiel-Tison, evaluation every 3 months is more than enough. After the examination is complete, the examiner can sum up the findings under these headings:
- Head growth
- Neurobehavior
- Neurosensory
- *Neuromotor:*
    - Hypertonia or hypotonia in upper limbs, lower limbs, or axis
    - Reflexes
    - Motor milestones

At the end of 12 months, three patterns emerge:
1. Babies who have shown normal development at all examinations in the first year
2. Babies who show tone abnormalities and developmental delay and are definitely brain damaged
3. Babies who show abnormal development at 3 and 6 months, start normalizing at 9 months and are normal at 12 months. It is this group of transient neurological abnormalities[5] which is of great interest to us, and had not been recognized in the past. These infants have been reported to have significantly poor scores in tests of cognitive function than their unaffected peers and are likely to present with learning difficulties in

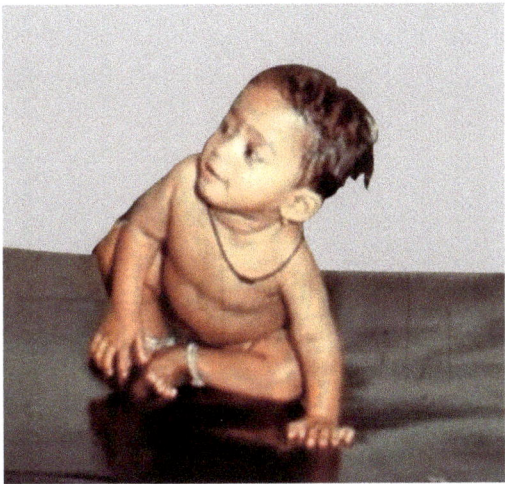

Fig. 9: Lateral propping reflex.

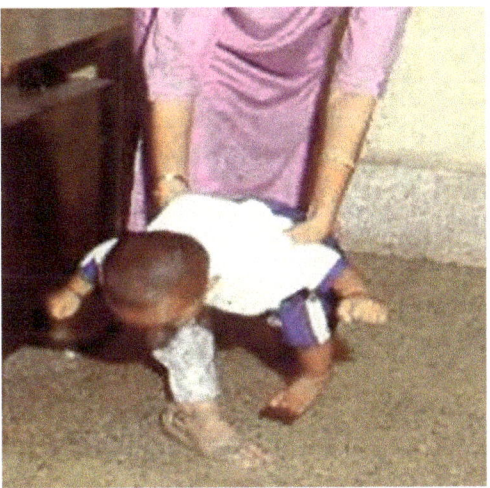

Fig. 10: Parachute reflex.

school, as they grow older. The learning difficulties appear much later, by which time the transient neurological abnormalities have been forgotten.

For planning interventional therapy by an occupational therapist, we classified our patients in two groups—those with tone abnormalities and those with developmental delay. The longitudinal pattern in tone abnormalities is more significant than scattered isolated anomalies. Babies with generalized hypertonia showed a greater risk (relative risk 5.03) for developing cerebral palsy than any other type. **Figure 6** shows abnormal hypertonia of neck extensor muscles. **Figure 11** shows a spastic child "toe-walking."

Development was considered delayed if partial head control had not appeared by 3 months, momentary sitting when pulled to sit at 6 months, creeping by 9 months and walking sideways along furniture at 12 months, and

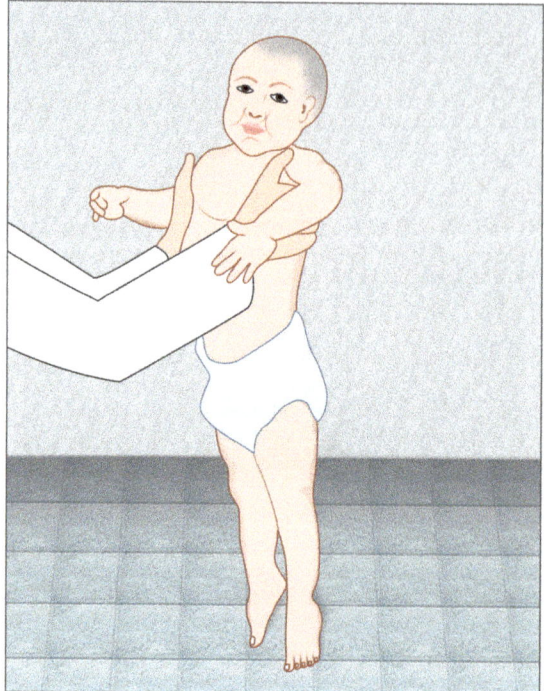

Fig. 11: Spastic infant "toe walking."

independent walking by 18 months. Postural reactions such as lateral propping should appear by 7 months and parachute reaction by 9 months. When infants with developmental delay were referred for testing with DASII, they were also found to be delayed on the motor scale.

This method of neurological assessment does not replace developmental tests and it does not take mental development into consideration. As reported by us,[5] it is a good screening test to decide which of the babies should be referred for the more elaborate developmental tests. We tested a group of high-risk infants with the DASII as well as with Amiel-Tison method. The Amiel-Tison method had greater sensitivity for picking up delayed motor development at 3, 6, and 9 months than the DASII, but lost this advantage at 12 months.[6]

Amiel-Tison has given ranges of the different angles. The question was whether angles described in Caucasian, French infants would be the same as Indian infants. Hence, we measured the various angles in 100 normal infants attending the Well Baby Clinic using a goniometer for accuracy.[7] We calculated the mean and standard deviation of each angle measured till the age of 12 months. The angles were pretty similar to the ranges described by Amiel-Tison. We have devised a special form for the neurological assessment of infants in the first year of life **(Annexure I)**.

The main drawback of this method is that it does not take mental development into consideration, and hence does not replace developmental tests.

It is a good screening test to identify infants who need occupational therapy and to decide which infants need to be referred for the more elaborate developmental tests. We have reported that if the 3-month assessment by Amiel-Tison was normal, the predictive value for a normal 12-month motor development was 93.6%.[8]

TRANSIENT TONE ABNORMALITIES

A syndrome of transiently abnormal neurologic signs was described by Drillen in preterm infants. She found neuromotor abnormalities in 40% of LBW infants, which resolved by 1 year. She followed them up to school age and found that they had a normal IQ. Amiel-Tison defined transient tone abnormalities (TTA), as those which are present in early infancy, but disappear by the end of 1 year. However, she questioned the assumption that these abnormalities are innocuous and found that these children had school difficulties. In the Pune Low Birth Study, 40.5% infants had tone abnormalities at 6 months, out of these 20.7% had hypertonia, 29.8% had hypotonia, and the remaining had minor tone abnormalities. About 87% of this group with tone abnormalities, started normalizing at 9 months and had no tone abnormalities at 1 year. All these infants were recalled at 5 years and an IQ was done.[9] The mean IQ of the TTA group was 98.5 ± 12.4, well within the normal range. **Figure 12** shows the transient nature of tone abnormalities in extremely low birth weight (ELBW) infants reported by us.[10] Hence, it is important not to make a diagnosis of cerebral palsy before 1 year, because many of these tone abnormalities are transient.[11]

QUALITATIVE AND QUANTITATIVE ASSESSMENT

Preterm infants develop differently and with more variability than full-term infants. The lower the gestational age, more the variability. Early assessments

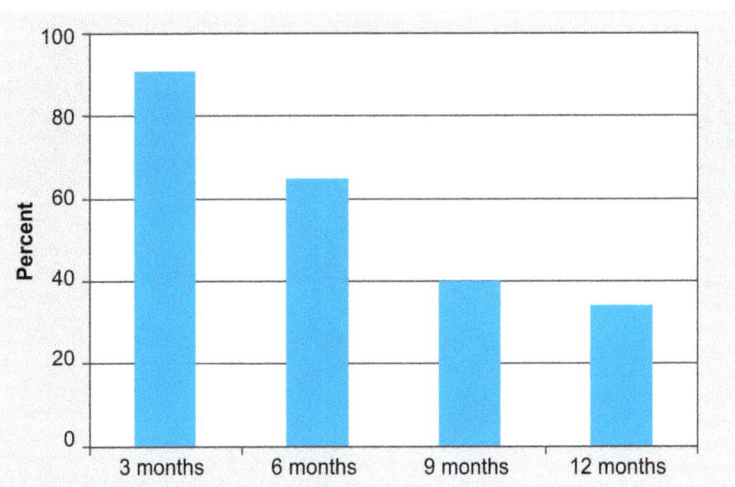

Fig. 12: Transient tone abnormalities in extremely low birth weight (ELBW) infants.

may not necessarily be predictive of final outcome, and the severity of the neurologic insult may not correlate with the final outcome. The true course will be determined only by a sequential examination over a period of time.

Often infants and children achieve an age-appropriate motor skill, but it appears abnormal in quality. Persistence of abnormality in movements may indicate a muscle tone disorder and needs further evaluation. Quality deviations are commonly seen in the following:

- *Rolling:*
  - Rolls only in one direction
  - By hyperextending trunk and neck to initiate and complete a roll
  - Getting arms caught under body when rolling from supine to prone position
- *Sitting:*
  - In a "W" fashion only **(Fig. 13)**
  - Rigidity with an inability to reach above head or across midline without losing balance
  - Arching out in a sitting position and falling backward
- *Crawling:*
  - On stomach only, rather than on hands and feet
  - With legs stiff, unable to crawl using legs reciprocally
  - On fisted hands
  - Using an asymmetric pattern
- *Pulling to stand:*
  - Using arm strength only without pushing off with legs
  - Showing stiffness, needs excessive effort
- *Standing:*
  - On toes most of the time
  - With excessive rigidity about the knees

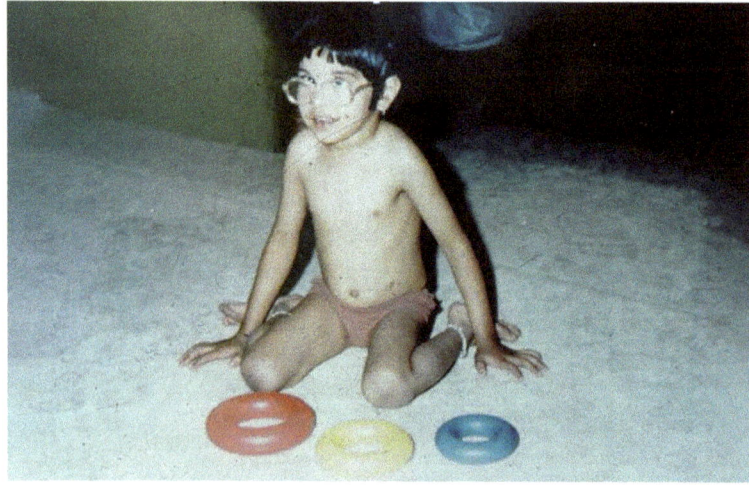

Fig. 13: "W" sitting.

- *Cruising:*
  - In one direction only
  - With legs stiff at knee
- Reaching, using hand preference before 2 years of age
- Grasping without ability to pick up objects with age-appropriate skills

PRECOCIOUS ACHIEVEMENT OF MOTOR MILESTONES

- Children with significant extensor hypertonicity demonstrate rolling skills and standing before expected time. These children may stand holding the sides of the crib, roll from prone to supine at 2 months.
- Precocious skills result from abnormal quality of muscle tone. These will then interfere with normal progress of specific motor skills.
- Explaining to the parents why these abnormal skills should not be encouraged is often difficult, since they are proud of their child's "precocious" development. Explaining the normal sequence of gross motor skills (crawling should precede walking) may help.

DEVELOPMENTAL TESTS

The developmental tests mainly measure the behavior of infants and children in four major fields.

Motor Behavior
This is of main interest to the physician because it has neurologic implications.

Adaptive Behavior
This includes sensorimotor coordination, manipulation, and exploitation of objects and resourcefulness in utilizing past experiences for adjusting to new experiences. It is the best index of inherent capabilities.

Language
It includes vocalization, facial and manual cues indicating wants, as well as understanding of expression of others.

Personal Social Behavior
It has a much wider variation because it depends largely on culture and environment, but its expression is also a function of neurologic maturity.

Table 1 gives the summary of developmental tests.

Ages and Stages Questionnaire
The Ages and Stages Questionnaire (ASQ) is a parent-completed, child development screening test with 19 questionnaires ranging from 4 to 60 months that are identical in format and organized into five item domains (communication, gross motor, fine motor, problem solving, and personal social). Questions can be answered by parents with 7th grade education.

TABLE 1: Summary of developmental tests.

Test	Age	Assessment	Development index	Usefulness	Limitation
1. Ages and Stages Questionnaire Screening Test (ASQ)	4–60 months	Parent completed questionnaire. 19 age-specific questions. Gross motor, fine motor, communication, problem solving, personal social (pass, fail)	Quantitative sensitivity, specificity moderate to high	Can be used as a screening test in a well-baby clinic	Depends on intelligence and observations of the parents
2. Trivandrum Development Screening Chart (TDSC)	0–2 years	17 items from the Bayley scales are used, motor and mental items	Sensitivity, specificity moderate	Can be used as a screening test in a well-baby clinic	DDST used as a gold standard, which in itself is a screening test
3. Denver Development Screening Test (DDSTII)	0–30 months	Motor behavior. Adaptive behavior, personal, and social behavior, language development, risk category (normal, questionable, abnormal)	Quantitative, low-to-moderate sensitivity, specificity	For use in a busy clinic	Misses mild delay resulting in under referrals
4. Development Assessment Scale for Indian Infants (DASII) Adaptation of Bayley II Scales of Infant Development	0–30 months	Mental (163 items) Motor (67 items) Considered to be Gold Standard	MeQ ≥85 normal MoQ ≥85 normal 70-84 delayed development <70 retardation	Confirmatory test after screening tests have identified delay	Needs a trained psychologist and a sound proof room and a special kit
5. Bayley III Much longer test, takes 30 minutes for children <13 months and 50 minutes >13months	16 days to 42 months	Covers cognitive, language, fine, and gross motor and socioemotional development	Higher scores compared to Bayley II	Needs further validation before use in Indian children	Gives much higher scores hence may lead to under referral

For those with low-literacy level, it can be administered as an interview. Parents indicate "yes," "sometimes," or "not yet." The ASQ needs 15 minutes to complete and 2-3 minutes to score. It has moderate-to-high sensitivity and specificity. Juneja et al. have used a Hindi translation of the test with good results.

Trivandrum Development Screening Test

It is a community-based neurodevelopmental screening test. It comprises 17 simple items selected from the 230 items of the Baroda norms. The gold standard used for calculating the sensitivity (66%) and specificity (78%) of this test was the Denver Development Screening Test (DDST). There are many reports which question the validity of the DDST itself, and feel that DDST is not a very sensitive test and can miss many cases of mild development delay.

Denver Developmental Screening Test (1992)

This test is a screening test of cognitive and behavioral problems in the age group of 0-6 years. Tasks are grouped into four categories (fine motor skills, gross motor skills, social contact, and language). In this test, a subject's performance against the regular age distribution is noted. This test is widely used all over the world. But it has been criticized for being unreliable in predicting less severe or specific problems in children, resulting in under referrals. The test depicts in graphic form the ages at which 25, 50, 75, and 90% of children performed from birth to 6 years. It enables the examiner to visualize at any age how a child's development compares with that of other children.

Developmental Assessment Scale for Indian Infants (DASII)

The Bayley scales was standardized by Phatak for Indian Infants. This test consists of 163 mental items and 67 motor items. Both the scales express the child's performance by the number of items passed by the child. A DQ > 85 is considered as normal. The test must be administered by a trained psychologist, it needs a special kit and must be ideally performed in a soundproof room. This test is considered as the gold standard for assessing development (*See* **Chapter 6B**).

Bayley III

A new and much longer version of the Bayley scales, it covers the age group of 16 days to 42 months. It covers five domains—language, cognitive, fine and gross motor, and socioemotional. It takes 30 minutes administration time for children below 13 months and 50 minutes for children 13 months and above. This test has been criticized because it yields higher than expected scores which may lead to under referrals (*See* **Chapter 6C**).

Baroda Development Screening Test

This test was designed for the use of community health workers for a door-to-door survey in the Baroda slums. This test is also based on the Baroda norms. It has 22 motor items and 31 mental items using commonly available material.

The items are arranged sequentially according to their 97% pass placement. This means that 97% of the children will pass that item at that particular age. A checklist is prepared and a child who fails the items in his or her age group is considered delayed.

Portage Early Education Program

The Portage Early Education Program incorporating the Wessex revised language checklist originated in the USA and has been widely used in the UK as well. The greatest advantage of this test is that it is not only a diagnostic test, but also has an inbuilt therapeutic or remedial program. This is the only developmental test which has this added advantage.

It assesses six areas of development, viz., infant stimulation, language, socialization, self-help, and motor and cognitive abilities. It was started as a community-based program. The field worker assesses the child at home and then trains the parents to teach the child whichever activity he or she could not perform during the test. Special activity cards are given to the parents which break up the activity into small teachable steps. The field worker then monitors the progress of the child by weekly visits. There is a Yes/No scoring for the skill, and a column for the date on which the child masters the skill.

This is a concise list of all the tests that are commonly used in India to assess the development of high-risk children. Every pediatrician who is involved in the follow-up of high-risk children must familiarize himself or herself with at least one of these tests.

INVESTIGATIONS

Investigations aim at establishing a possible etiology underlying the child's specific developmental delay. The etiology may or may not be apparent at the end of the clinical examination. Determining the underlying etiology is important for many reasons. It imparts an understanding of the pathogenesis to the family, answering their "need to know why." In genetic conditions, it has implications regarding recurrence risk.

Low Cognitive Abilities and Borderline Intelligence

It has become increasingly evident that "high-risk" infants experience significant functional learning impairments that become apparent at school age. Learning problems affect the ability of the "high-risk" infant to learn mathematics, reading, writing, and other academic subjects. The incidence of "slow learners" (IQ 70–84) has been variously reported from 14 to 27% in very low birth weight (VLBW) infants **(Fig. 14)**.

"Borderline intelligence" or low cognitive abilities are defined as functioning below average, but not in the range of mental retardation. This includes the children, referred to as "slow learners," whose IQ ranges between 70 and 84. Frequently, it goes undiagnosed except for casual observation of

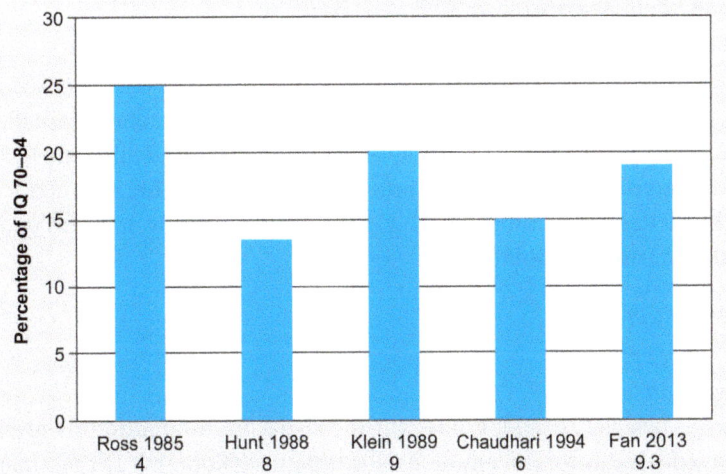

Fig. 14: Incidence of "borderline intelligence" in very low birth weight (VLBW) infants.

a child who appears less bright than his siblings or because of school failure. Although the functioning of the child is almost appropriate for age, the child has an over-reliance on repetition or rote learning. These children often express a preference for familiar routine. The level of concern expressed by the parents depends on cultural and familial expectations. Families with a strong emphasis on high academic achievements are likely to express anxiety with the learning rate or slow achievement of the child. They often attribute it to slowness and laziness. Diagnosis helps in acceptance and reduces the pressure on the child. Families who are not very educated and not very "achievement oriented," may find it easier to integrate this child. Teachers will also be more sensitive to the child's needs when the problem is explained to them. The child may ultimately be shifted to a special school when it becomes obvious that he or she cannot cope in a normal school. Environmental stimulation also plays a major role in the performance of these children.

Intelligence Tests

Stanford–Binet Intelligence Scale

Age: 2.0–18 years

Time approximately 30 minutes:

This test is commonly used in school children to determine the IQ. It measures different intellectual abilities such as language skills, immediate and sustained memory, abstract thinking, reasoning, and numerical reasoning. An Indian adaptation in Hindi by Kulshrestha and in Marathi and Kannada by Kamat is available. Since progress in intellectual development is so rapid between 2 and 4 years, it proceeds by ½ year intervals and later on by yearly intervals. It requires a highly trained psychologist who needs to record the subject's responses along with personality, activity level, self-confidence, and concentration.

Wechsler Intelligence Scale for Children (WISC-R)

Age: 5–15 years
Time approximately 40 minutes

It measures intelligence on a point scale measure, and an Indian adaptation by Bhat is available. It yields a verbal IQ, performance IQ, and full scale IQ. Both speed and performance are taken into account while scoring arithmetic, digit span, block design, picture assembly, and object assembly. It is also good for detecting learning disabilities.

Bender-Gestalt Test

Age: 5–11 years
No time limit

This test is basically used for detecting the visual-motor maturation level and also provides indicators for emotional disturbances (Koppitz). The test material consists of: (1) Nine figures each on a different card, (2) a response sheet 8.5" × 11", and (3) a stop watch. The child is given the 9 cards one by one, is asked to copy the design. The time taken is also noted. It is a subjective test, and formal schooling improves the performance.

Draw a Man Test (Phatak)
Human Figure Drawing (Koppitz)

Age: 4–15 years

The child is asked to draw a complete picture of a man using paper and pencil. This drawing is later analyzed to judge his or her intelligence and his or her mental and emotional setup. The technique by which the IQ is derived is called Draw a Man Test (Goodenough, 1926). This is standardized for Indian children by Phatak. It gives a very wide range of IQ. The same protocol can be used as a projective technique and is called Human Figure Drawing (Koppitz). Three main aspects of the drawing are analyzed, viz., quality signs, special features, and omissions. There are 30 emotional indicators and if two or more indicators are present, the child is considered to be emotionally disturbed.

Raval's Social Maturity Scale

Age: 0–10 years
Time approximately 15 minutes

It is in the form of an interview of the mother or caregiver. The interview is different for urban and rural children. The interviewer is not allowed to use his or her own observations but has to record what the mother says. This is the main drawback of this test. This scale is very useful for assessing children with cerebral palsy. In these children, the mental faculties may be quite good but the child performs poorly on the development scale due to the motor handicap. In such a situation, the information regarding the child's development provided by the mother is very useful.

Early identification of children with developmental delays or disabilities can lead to early intervention and treatment and lessen its impact on the child.

Developmental surveillance is an important way of detecting developmental delays. The neonatologist should be skilled in the use of screening techniques, carefully listen to parental concerns, and create links with available resources in the community.

REFERENCES

1. Chaudhari S. In: Guha D (Ed). Guha's Neonatology, 3rd edition. New Delhi: Jaypee Brothers Medical Publishers; 2005. pp. 1169-77.
2. Chaudhari S, Otiv M, Hoge M, Pandit A, Mote A. Growth and sexual maturation of low birth weight infants at early adolescence. Indian Pediatr. 2008;45(3):191-8.
3. Chaudhari S, Otiv M, Chitale A, Hoge M, Pandit A, Mote A. Biology versus environment in low birth weight children. Indian Pediatr. 2005;42(8):763-70.
4. Amiel-Tison C. A method for neurological evaluation with first year of life. Current Problems in Pediatrics VII No 1. Chicago: Year Book Medical Publishers; 1976. pp. 1-50.
5. Chaudhari S, Bhalerao M, Chitale A, Patil B, Pandit A, Hoge M. Transient tone abnormalities in "High Risk" infants and cognitive outcome at five years. Indian Pediatr. 2010;47(11):931-5.
6. Chaudhari S, Shinde SV, Barve, Dixit HS, Pandit A. A longitudinal follow-up of neurodevelopment of high risk newborns: a comparison of Amiel-Tison's method with Bayley scales of infant development. Indian Pediatr. 1990;27(8):799-802.
7. Chaudhari S, Deo B. Neurodevelopmental assessment in the first year with emphasis on evolution of tone. Indian Pediatr. 2006;43(6):527-34.
8. Chaudhari S, Kulkarni S, Pandit A, Koundinya. Neurological assessment at three months as a predictor for developmental in high risk infants. Indian Pediatr. 1993;30(4):528-31.
9. Chaudhari S, Bhalerao MR, Chitale A, Pandit AN, Nene U. Pune low birth weight study: a six-year follow up. Indian Pediatr. 1999;36(7):669-76.
10. Tagare A, Chaudhari S, Kadam S, Vaidya UV, Pandit A. Mortality and morbidity in extremely low birth (ELBW) infants in neonatal intensive care unit. Indian J Pediatr. 2013;80(1):16-20.
11. Bernbaum I, Hoffman-Williamson M. Primary care of the preterm infant. St Louis: Mosby Yearbook; 1991.

Developmental Assessment Scales for Indian Infants (DASII)

CHAPTER 6B

Bindu Patni

INTRODUCTION

A developmental assessment is a structured evaluation of the child's development and a comprehensive assessment needs to cover the key domains—physical, social, emotional, moral, and intellectual.[1]

Developmental assessments are useful to assess a young child's current skills relative to where they should be compared to a typical child's development. They are structured systems of observation. Standardized tools have the benefit of being easy to implement. Most developmental tests attempt to measure the unfolding of the developmental sequence. The development of abilities in the first 2 years of life is a combination of sensory, motor, and mental skills. The focus of assessment largely revolves around domains such as physical growth, gross and fine motor development, social emotional development, cognitive development, and personal social development.

The appropriate choice of a tool for assessment depends on the purpose of assessment. Developmental assessment may be for screening purposes, in order to identify at-risk babies for a particular problem and to start early intervention. Most screening tools are brief checklists of red flag signs. More detailed diagnostic assessment may be needed for classification and understanding the nature and severity of the problem and to identify special needs. An assessment may also be carried out to evaluate efficacy of treatment and intervention.

With better neonatal care over the years, the survival rate of high-risk infants has resulted in a large number of infants needing surveillance, screening, and assessment for early detection and early intervention procedures. In our country, routine formal screening of all babies is neither feasible nor cost-effective. However, screening should be done in all high-risk infants at age as early as 3–6 months, and referred for detailed evaluation, if indicated.

Developmental assessment of infants poses a lot of challenges due to various reasons. A cooperative child is the crux of successful infant testing. Motivating the child for optimum performance is a skill that needs to be developed. The entire testing process has to be a guided play activity for the child and an opportunity to observe performance for the tester. A baby's mental status and interest in the test material is easily affected by the baby's mood, hunger, requirement of sleep, and optimum physical health. Sometimes, it is observed that children show persistent interest in certain toy materials even after the observation is complete. At other times, they have a desire to possess a particular material, and they want to take it home. Some babies react with fear to certain test items such as a doll. Sometimes, it is difficult to complete a satisfactory assessment in a single session due to these factors.

Parental interference is another challenge that needs to be handled.[2] Anxiety about the child's performance and spontaneous attempts at helping the child perform, can affect the reliability of a performance. There are times when a parent's help may be sought to stimulate or evoke certain responses from the child or to motivate the child to do certain activities, especially on the motor scale. However, these have to be controlled by the examiner and the parent should help only when requested to. Free play between the mother and the child before or after the assessment may be utilized to credit certain items which are observational.

As in any standardized assessment, developmental assessment tools also require a standardized procedure to be meticulously followed during testing. Using the standardized test material as well as standardized administration procedures, is of utmost importance to obtain reliable and valid results. Often the test materials in a developmental tool look like common toys, but should never be replaced with anything except the materials provided in the test kit **(Fig. 1)**.

Most developmental assessment tests, except some of the screening tests, require some training for administration. Interpretation of the test scores requires knowledge of psychometric assessment. Diagnosis of developmental delay should be made with caution, only after considering all the factors that could have affected the overall scores. Some of the severely affected babies

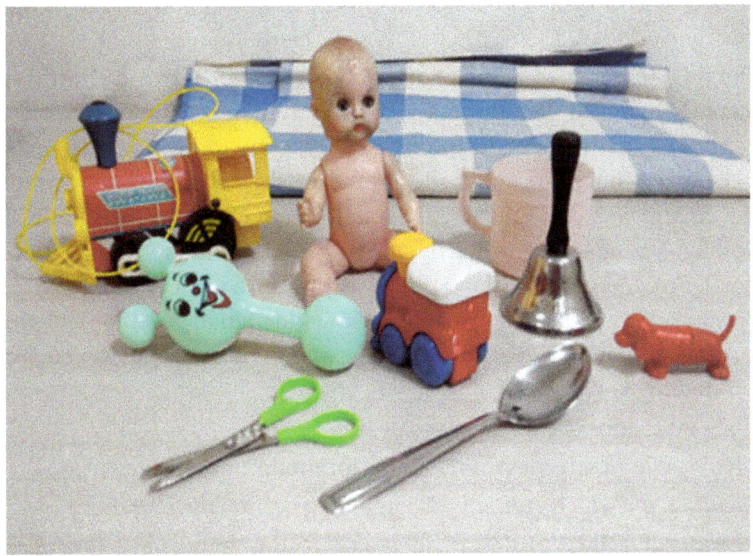

Fig. 1: Developmental Assessment Scales for Indian Infants (DASII) kit.

may not be able to perform on a developmental test, and assessment can be postponed and carried out after some intervention is initiated.

We need to remember that assessment is not an end in itself. It is a means to an end, which is, planning an intervention program. The work of a pediatrician or therapist does not end with an assessment but really begins once the assessment results are obtained.

A significant developmental delay is diagnosed when there is 25% delay in functioning or if the score falls 2 standard deviations below average. A global developmental delay is diagnosed when the performance is low in two or more domains within the scale. In case of a preterm baby, standard scores or composite scores must be calculated using corrected age till the age of 2 years.

A word of caution is needed here as the score obtained on a developmental scale should never be used for prediction of adult intelligence levels. A developmental assessment tool attempts to assess the current level of functioning or developmental status, as at this age level, the skills are still unfolding and are a product of emerging sensorimotor, socioemotional development.

Two useful tools for the infant's developmental assessment are both derived from the original work of Nancy Bayley. The Bayley Scales of Infant Development (BSID) was first published in USA in 1969. Developmental Assessment Scales for Indian Infants (DASII) is considered as a gold standard for assessment of Indian babies.

The original work was done by Dr Pramila Phatak and first published as Baroda norms in 1970, which was based on research form 1961 by Nancy Bayley. This publication was based on longitudinal testing of normal healthy babies from 1 to 30 months. A total of 4,100 records were analyzed and published as Baroda norms. In 1987, a second edition of the document was published by Dr Pramila Phatak. The initial work was carried out at the MS University, Vadodara.[3]

Her final publication involved revision of these 1970 Baroda norms using indigenous material. The difficulty in procurement of the testing kit from USA and the expense involved, prompted her to use indigenous test material. This also made it a more culturally appropriate testing kit which was locally produced and was cost-effective. The major data collection was done at MS University, Vadodara,[4] and partly at Child Development Unit at the KEM Hospital, Pune.[5] This combined data was published as DASII in 1996.[5] This publication also included her work on motor and mental development profiles of normal babies of 1 to 30 months of age and their use as reference profiles in therapeutic work.[6]

The DASII consists of two subscales:
- *Motor scale* which contains 67 items for motor development
- *Mental scale* which contains 163 items for mental development

The motor scale is further divided after factor analysis into the following clusters as shown in **Box 1**.

BOX 1: Motor and mental clusters.

Motor Clusters
- Neck control (7 items)
- Body control (23 items)
- Locomotion 1 (10 items)
- Locomotion 2 (13 items)
- Manipulation (14 items)

Mental Clusters
- Visual cognizance (25 items)
- Auditory cognizance (7 items)
- Reaching manipulation and exploring (36 items)
- Memory (11 items)
- Social interaction and imitative behavior (22 items)
- Language 1 (11 items)
- Language 2 (18 items)
- Understanding of relationship (18 items)
- Differentiation by use, shapes, and movements (8 items)
- Manual dexterity (7 items)

MOTOR CLUSTERS

Motor items cover both gross motor and fine motor skill development.
- *Neck control (7 items)*: This cluster assesses stages in head holding and neck control.
- *Body control (23 items)*: This cluster covers the child's development from supine to erect posture. It requires observations of hand and leg movements, rolling over, and development of sitting and coming to standing posture.
- *Locomotion 1 (10 items)*: This includes basic locomotive skills including prewalking progression, crawling, walking with support, and independent walking.
- *Locomotion 2 (13 items)*: This cluster includes locomotive skills such as climbing, jumping, and skipping.
- *Manipulation (14 items)*: This cluster records manipulatory behaviors such as reaching, picking up things, handling and manipulating objects, putting, or throwing them in a directed manner. It includes assessment of grasp from palmar to radial, digital to pincer.

MENTAL CLUSTERS

Mental clusters cover a variety of developmental domains including cognition, memory, language, and rudimentary screening of hearing and vision.
- *Visual cognizance (25 items)*: This cluster includes items measuring visual fixation and visual pursuit of objects. It uses a variety of stimuli such as a moving person, torchlight, red ring, and a yellow pencil. It helps in screening very early visual deficits which prevent the baby from fixating or following moving objects. This kind of early screening helps for further referral in case of inconsistent responses **(Fig. 2)**.
- *Auditory cognizance (7 items)*: This is also a useful procedure for early screening of auditory deficits. Various auditory stimuli such as sound of a

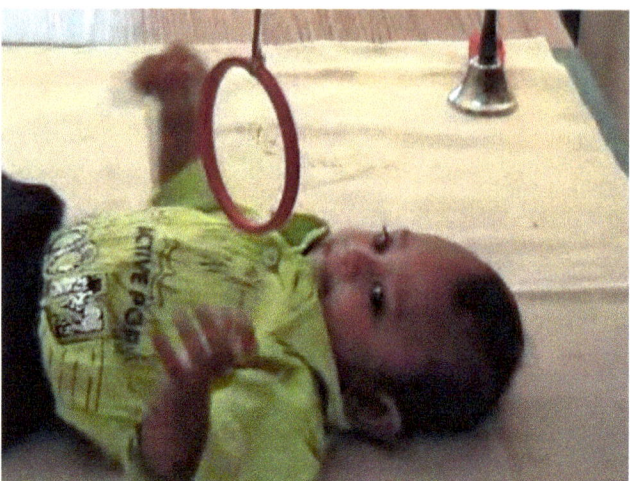

Fig. 2: Visual cognizance—red ring.

bell, rattle, light switch, and human voice are utilized to assess the baby's hearing acuity. It also helps in assessment of ability for sound localization. The stimuli are presented on either side of the head to assess bilateral functioning and helps in early referral in case of doubtful responses.

- *Reaching manipulation and exploring (36 items)*: This cluster assesses the child's awareness of objects in his surrounding and exploring them to meaningful manipulation. It covers skills such as voluntary reach for objects such as a red cube, to making a tower of eight cubes. Typically, babies go through a stage of mouthing objects. Excessive mouthing of test material that is offered sometimes hampers successful performance on an item.
- *Memory (11 items)*: These items assess development of object permanence and recognition of familiarity. The items range from recognition of his mother's face to finding a hidden object. Very restless and distracted babies often do not perform well on such memory items.
- *Social interaction and imitative behavior (22 items)*: This aspect of development is assessed with the help of social and imitative play with the child. The child's reaction to appreciation and imitative intent is assessed here. Social and imitative behavior is a very important learning tool in the baby's behavioral repertoire.
- *Language 1 (11 items)*: This cluster assesses vocalization, development of speech and communication. It includes vocalization of syllables, babbling, jargon, and use of gestures and words to communicate. It is important to assess the baby in its mother tongue and be familiar with the local baby language which is culturally appropriate.
- *Language 2 (18 items)*: This cluster includes receptive language, comprehension of spoken language, following verbal commands, and picture vocabulary. For example, the picture vocabulary item contains familiar objects from the baby's environment such as a dog, a cup, or a shoe.
- *Understanding of relationship (18 items)*: This cluster assesses baby's understanding of object relationship using objects such as a ring tied with

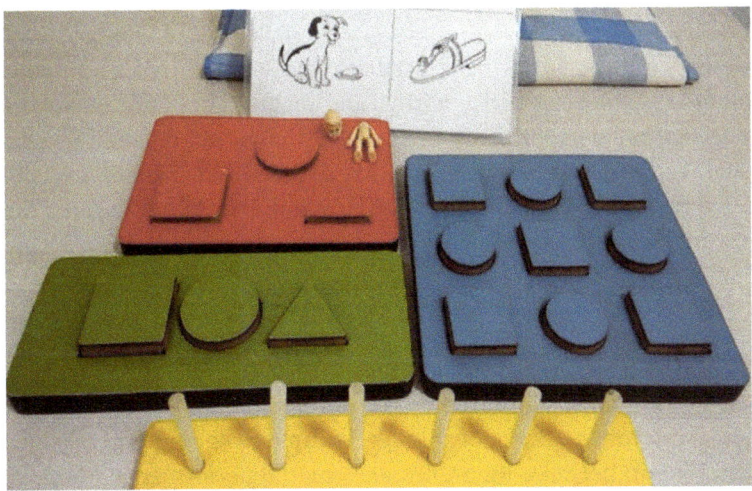

Fig. 3: *Understanding of relationship:* Form board and broken doll.

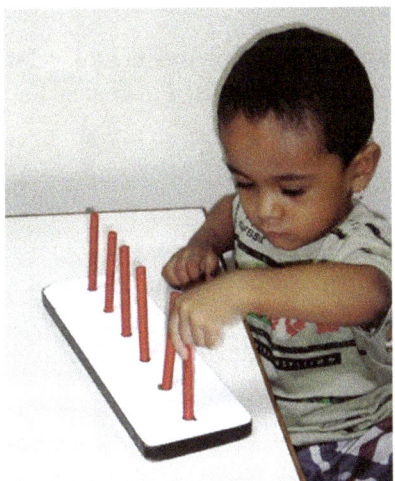

Fig. 4: Manual dexterity—peg board test.

a string or form boards with cutouts of shapes **(Fig. 3)**. Understanding body parts on a doll or mending a broken doll also involves understanding of part whole relationship. The baby has to fit a broken head of the doll in an appropriate position and at the appropriate joint on the torso. Understanding of prepositions is also under this cluster indicating understanding of spatial relationships. The baby is expected to understand words such as in, under, over, and behind.

- *Differentiation by use, shapes, and movements (8 items)*: This cluster includes items such as ringing a bell, scribbling on paper, imitating strokes on paper, and perceptual discrimination of objects like a plate, cup, box, etc.
- *Manual dexterity (7 items)*: This cluster includes some of the very few timed items which require speed of performance and finger dexterity. This includes use of pegboard and form boards **(Fig. 4)**.

STANDARDIZATION

The strength of the scale lies in the fact that it was standardized on a longitudinal sample of 513 babies certified as normal and healthy. They were assessed at the child development department and well baby clinic at Maharani Shantadevi Hospital, Vadodara. The data for the first 30 days of life of babies was based upon 155 records of 139 babies at KEM Hospital, Pune. They covered the age range from birth to 45 days.[7]

PSYCHOMETRIC PROPERTIES

Validity

The face validity was supported by the developmental validity in the trend of increasing mean scores of the age groups, as the age increased. The intercorrelation between the motor and mental performance of the scales ranges from 0.24 to 0.62.

Reliability

The median reliability index for motor and mental scales based on correlation between consecutive months is reported to be 0.88 for motor scale and 0.91 for mental scales.

ADMINISTRATION TIME

It takes about 30 minutes for babies below 1 year and 45 minutes to an hour for older babies. It is simultaneous but independent administration of the motor and mental items. A baby is administered items placed around his developmental level till 10 consecutive pass or fail on either side is achieved.

ADMINISTRATION PROCEDURE

Administering the DASII scale requires training and should be done by a certified DASII trainer. It requires a quiet soundproof room with appropriate furniture made to specification given in the test manual **(Fig. 5)**. This should ensure comfortable seating and handling of the test materials offered to the child.

Motor and mental items are administered simultaneously during the testing. In our experience, it may be better to start with the motor items for a toddler above the age of 2 years, who may be allowed to run around and explore the testing room while observing some of his motor skills. For younger babies, it is advisable to administer the motor items which require handling of the baby during the latter part of the testing session. Sometimes, a stranger touching or carrying the baby may upset the baby and result in crying and result in noncooperation. Babies who are also undergoing physiotherapy or occupational therapy may have negative associations about clinicians touching them. However, most of the time, the motor and mental items are intermingled during a typical assessment.

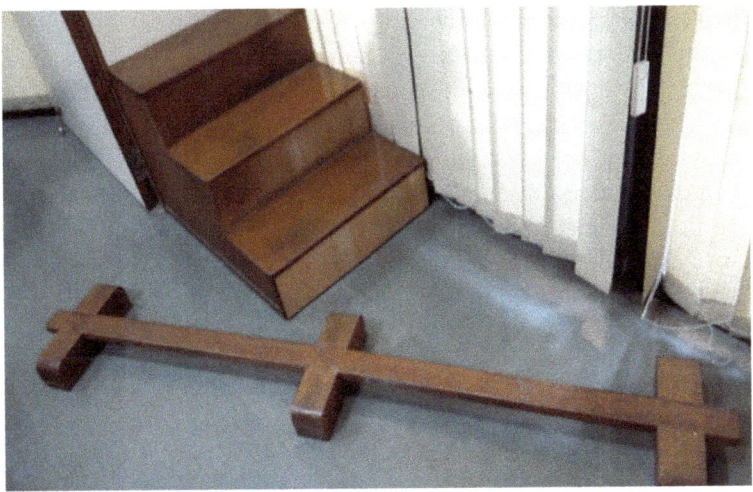

Fig. 5: Furniture needed for motor scale.

SCORING

It is a point scale with items arranged in order of increasing difficulty. Total raw score on each scale is converted into motor age and mental age, respectively. The reference point that is usually considered is 50% pass level age placement. However, the records also report 3% and 97% pass level age placements as limits of performance of each item. A Developmental Quotient (DQ) can be calculated by comparing the developmental age with the chronological age. For example, Motor DQ = Mo Age/chronological age × 100. Deviation quotient equivalent to total raw score as well as percentile ranks of deviation quotients are also available. Each content cluster obtains a percentile score which can be plotted as motor performance profile and mental performance profile. These profiles of mental and motor performance are very useful for diagnostic formulations.[4]

Profile Analysis of the Cluster Scores provides more clinically useful information related to early developmental problems, helping us to target early intervention program to more specific areas of weakness. It also aids in differential diagnosis with different profiles for various developmental disabilities.[4]

Our experience shows certain profiles to be typical in certain diagnostic groups. Typically, a child with cerebral palsy will perform better on the mental clusters than on the motor clusters. Within the mental clusters, he will show better skills on language comprehension, memory, and social imitative behaviors. A child with Down's syndrome will show some motor delay, especially fine motor skills, but very good scores on social imitative behavior. He may have poor scores on other mental clusters.

The discrepancy between verbal and nonverbal mental clusters, average score on motor scale, along with inconsistent response to auditory stimuli and spoken language may help diagnose mild hearing impairment in toddlers.

Toddlers with early signs of autism are more likely to show average motor development score with scattered performance on the mental scale. They also exhibit poor social imitative score and low performance on the language clusters. They have often been observed to show very good understanding of relationships, high speed for manual dexterity items such as peg boards, and form boards with shape discrimination. They often show fixation or fascination with certain test materials which also raises doubts about early signs of autism. Thus, with an experienced clinician, the DASII scale can be a very useful diagnostic tool, in addition to being a gold standard for developmental assessment.

REFERENCES

1. Wright JD. International Encyclopaedia of Social and Behavioral Sciences, 2nd edition. Amsterdam: Elsevier; 2015.
2. Patni B. Developmental assessment scales for Indian infants. Indian J Pract Pediatr. 2012;14(4):409-12.
3. Phatak P. Motor and mental development profiles of normal babies 1–30 months and use of reference profiles in therapeutic work. Indian J Clinical Psychol. 1995;22:36-42.
4. Phatak P, Barve S, Pandit AN. Motor and mental development of normal babies (1–45 days). Indian Pediatr. 1984;21:521-8.
5. Phatak P, Misra N. Developmental assessment scales for Indian infants (DASII) 1–30 months: Revision of Baroda norms with indigenous material. Psychol Stud. 1996;41:55-6.
6. Phatak P. Mental and motor growth of Indian babies (1–30 months): Final report, 2nd edition. Baroda: Department of Child Development, Faculty of Home Science, MS University of Baroda; 1987.

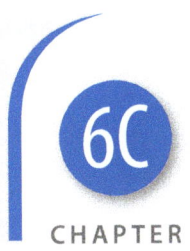

CHAPTER 6C

Bayley Scales of Infant and Toddler Development: Third Edition (Bayley III)

Bindu Patni

INTRODUCTION

The Bayley Scales of Infant and Toddler Development-Bayley III is a revision of the Bayley Scales of Infant Development, 2nd edition. This revision was done to improve the quality and to enhance the utility of the instrument. This is an individually administered scale that assesses developmental functioning of infants and young children, 1 –42 months of age. The primary purpose of the scale is identification of children with developmental delay and planning of intervention. The main difference in the second revision is extension of the scale up to 42 months to include toddler assessments.[1]

The Bayley III consists of the following three subscales:
1. Cognitive scale
2. Language scale
3. Motor scale

The language scale is further divided into: Receptive communication and expressive communication subtests. The separation of the language scale was introduced in this revision.

The motor scale is further divided into: Fine motor and gross motor subtests **(Box 1)**. The Bayley III test material is shown in **Figure 1**.

COGNITIVE SCALE

The cognitive scale is composed of 91 items which assesses attention to novelty, habituation, sensory motor development, and problem-solving. It also includes items assessing object relatedness, concept formation, number concepts and counting, and memory.

There is a very useful inclusion of items involving children's play activity. The cognitive scale incorporates items ranging from solitary non-relational play to social fantasy play. It is postulated that play activity promotes cognitive

BOX 1: Subscales of Bayley III.

- Cognitive scale
- *Language scale:*
  – Receptive communication
  – Expressive communication
- *Motor scale:*
  – Gross motor
  – Fine motor

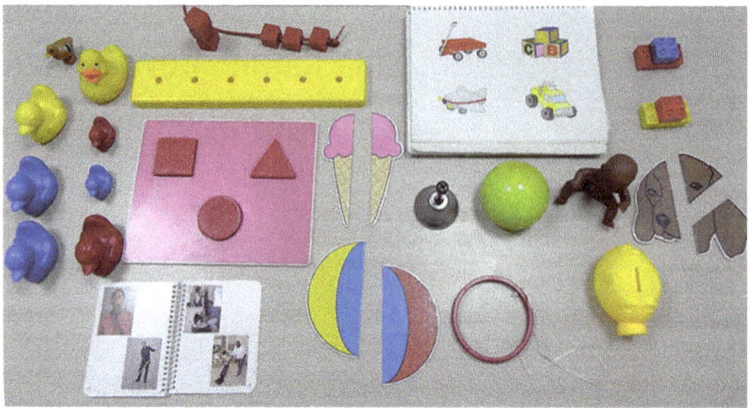

Fig. 1: Bayley III test material.

development. Development of play skills follows a sequence from interactive play, combination play, relational play, symbolic play, to pretend play. Thus, it becomes a useful measure of developmental sequence and developmental stage.

LANGUAGE SCALE

Receptive Communication Subtest

This scale comprises of 49 items, some of which assess auditory acuity. Other items focus on the child's ability to comprehend and respond to words and commands. There is an attempt to assess the child's ability for comprehension of spoken language. The items include assessment of understanding of plurals, prepositions, and the possessive.

Expressive Communication Subtest

This includes 48 items assessing ability to vocalize, starting with cooing and babbling. It goes on to measure the child's ability to make one word utterances, name pictures, name objects, name attributes such as color and size. It also assesses the ability to communicate needs and answer questions using multiple words and combine words and gestures.

There is criticism about the language scales that it contains significant cultural and linguistic biases, which preclude it from being appropriate for children from diverse backgrounds.[2] In our experience, the verbal items requiring certain grammar formation are not suitable to some of the Indian vernacular languages without modification.

MOTOR SCALE

Fine Motor Subtest

This includes 66 items that measure the infant's ability for coordinated eye movements and scanning of objects. It also assesses reaching and grasping of objects, hand skills, and response to tactile information.

Gross Motor Subtest

This includes 72 items that assess motor milestone development, static position, coordination, balance, including development of locomotion, and motor planning.

The Bayley III also has incorporated a Social Emotional Scale which is based on the Greenspan social emotional growth chart.[3]

Bayley III also includes an Adaptive Behavior Observation Inventory which is completed by interviewing the caregiver. This is an adaptation from the Adaptive Behavior Assessment Systems by Harrison and Oakland, 2003.[4]

STANDARDIZATION

The Bayley III was standardized on a sample of 1,700 babies between the ages of 16 days and 43 months 15 days.

PSYCHOMETRIC PROPERTIES

The overall average reliability coefficient of the Bayley III subtests ranges from 86 to 91.

ADMINISTRATION TIME

For children below 12 months, it takes about 30 minutes to complete the test. With children above the age of 12 months, it takes about 45–70 minutes.

SCORING

The total raw score is obtained for each subtest by counting the total number of items the child has received credit for. The raw scores are converted into scaled scores ranging from 1 to 19 with the mean of 10 and standard deviation 3. The other test scores available are composite scores, percentile ranks, and developmental age equivalents. It is possible to plot a profile of the scores using the scaled scores. For more detailed analysis, discrepancy comparisons are also available. **Table 1** gives a comparison between DASII and Bayley III.

As we can see both these scales are very similar in that both have evolved from the same developmental tool by Nancy Bayley. The essential aspects of the two scales are also similar. Both are individually administered scales with similar test materials. The grouping and classification of the items has evolved differently over the years with more recent standardizations.

DASII has the advantage of being a very widely used indigenous tool with norms based on Indian babies with test material that is definitely more culturally appropriate. Bayley III has the advantage of covering toddler age range up to 42 months, whereas DASII covers age range up to 30 months only. However, there are other equally useful and well-standardized tools available for assessment of babies beyond 30 months.

Bayley III is a robust tool with extensive research and stringent standardization procedures which is published in 2006 as compared to DASII

TABLE 1: Comparison of DASII and Bayley III.

DASII	Bayley III
• Based on BSID	• Based on BSID
• Norms based on Indian infants	• Norms based on foreign infants
• Individually administered scale	• Individually administered scale
• Requires trained personnel	• Requires trained personnel
• Requires around 1 hour to complete	• Requires around 1 hour to complete
• Indian adaptation	• American standardization
• Covers age range up to 30 months	• Covers age range up to 42 months
• Assessment divided into two domains—mental and motor	• Assessment divided into 5 domains
• Gives profile of performance based on 5 motor and 10 mental clusters	• Gives two optional scales, social, emotional and adaptive behavior
• Low cost	• Prohibitive cost
• No recent revision	• More recent revision
• Culturally appropriate items	• Culturally inappropriate
• Appropriate referrals	• Under referrals

(BSID: Bayley Scales of Infant Development; DASII: Developmental Assessment Scales for Indian Infants)

which is published in 1996. Having used both the scales for assessment of babies, it can be said that DASII is a more culturally appropriate tool. Some of the test materials such as picture vocabulary or language items are not directly translatable to Indian vernacular languages. While assessing infants below 3 years, the language of testing, i.e., baby's mother tongue is a very crucial aspect of rapport establishment and encouraging the baby to communicate and evaluating his utterances.

Many clinicians also suggest that Bayley III overestimates development and as such underestimates delay.[5] This may result in underdiagnosis of developmental delay. Another prohibitive factor about the Bayley III is the cost involved. This can be an enormous factor in reducing its popularity among users all over India.

Any robust developmental assessment should incorporate the following broad guidelines:
- It is very important to understand the parental concerns regarding the baby. A detailed interview with the parents and listening to their observations provides major clues for a meaningful assessment.
- It is imperative that we document a detailed developmental history and document all the prenatal, natal, and postnatal information which may be tied in with the findings of the assessment.
- We need to determine the purpose of a formal assessment and whether it will add to what we already know about the baby through other sources.
- We need to start with relationship building with the parent and family for a successful assessment and constructive follow-up.
- The psychologist conducting the assessment has to be open to listening rather than telling the parents at the initial stage.
- We need to fully explain the purpose of assessment at the outset and the result of assessment at the final stage.

- Including parents and family at all stages of assessment helps in making it a collaborative process and aids in long-term follow-up.

REFERENCES

1. Bayley N. Bayley Scales of Infant and Toddler Development. Technical Manual, 3rd edition. UK: Pearson Education Inc; 2006.
2. Test Review: Bayley III by Leadership Project, Columbia Univ. New York, 2013.
3. Greenspan SI. Greenspan Social Emotional Growth Chart: A Screening Questionnaire for Infants and Young Children. San Antonio: Harcourt Assessment; 2004.
4. Harrison PL, Oakland, T. Adaptive behaviour assessment system, 2nd edition. San Antonio: The Psychological Corporation; 2003.
5. Anderson PJ, De Luca CR, Hutchinson E, Gehan Roberts, Lex W Doyle; Victorian Infant Collaborative Group. Underestimation of developmental delay by the new Bayley III scale. Arch Pedi Adolesc Med. 2010;164:352-6.

Cerebral Palsy

Sudha Chaudhari

INTRODUCTION

Cerebral palsy (CP) is a permanent disorder of posture and movement due to a nonprogressive lesion of the developing brain, following an injury before, during, or after birth. There may be additional problems such as seizures or vision deficits, language disorders, intellectual disability (mental retardation), sensory processing, and perceptual disorders. These depend on the location of the brain injury. The surveillance of cerebral palsy in Europe (SCPE) group describes five key factors for defining CP: (1) an umbrella term, (2) permanent, but not unchanging, (3) disorder of movement and/or posture and motor function, (4) due to a nonprogressive lesion or abnormality, and (5) affecting the immature brain.[1]

Cerebral palsy is not necessarily associated with cognitive deficits. There is paucity of prevalence data of CP in India. Chauhan et al.[2] did a meta-analysis of studies on prevalence of CP and concluded that it was 2.95/1,000 children. In a follow-up study of 336 "high-risk" infants, we found that 4.8% developed CP, 3.3% had associated mental retardation.[3] CP can be classified according to tone, location, and severity.

TONE

- *Hypertonic*: Stiff, associated with spasticity **(Fig. 1)**
- *Hypotonic*: Floppy, joint hypermobility **(Fig. 2)**
- *Dystonic*: May be athetoid or ataxic

CHILDREN WITH ATHETOSIS

- May be floppy to begin with
- May have significant feeding problems
- May have persistence of newborn primitive reflexes
- Have difficulty in maintaining head and hands in midline
- Have difficulty in movements against gravity and tend to go from complete flexion to extension

CHILDREN WITH ATAXIA

- May be floppy to begin with
- Usually maintain midline skills, they lose control if they are tilted from the midline

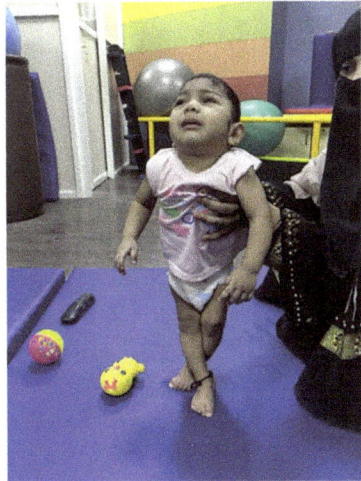 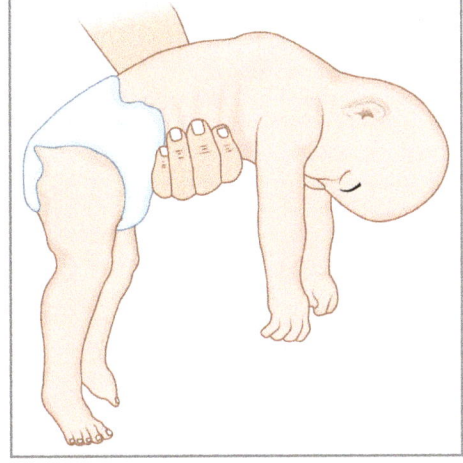

Fig. 1: Crossing of legs in a spastic infant.

Fig. 2: Hypotonic infant on horizontal suspension.

- They display tremors in hands and legs, which increase with effort and stress.
- Difficulty in grading movements
- Poor balance

TOPOGRAPHIC CLASSIFICATION (FIG. 3)

- *Quadriplegia*: Head, trunk, and all four limbs involved
- *Diplegia*: Legs more involved than arms.
- *Hemiplegia*: One side of the body is involved.
- *Monoplegia*: One limb is involved.
- *Triplegia*: Three limbs involved.

SEVERITY

- *Mild*: Ambulatory, independent in self-care
- *Moderate*: Ambulatory with assistive devices, may require some help in self-care
- *Severe*: Nonambulatory, need assistance in all self-care

It is mandatory to do a good developmental examination, at least every 3 months in a high-risk infant. Parents of high-risk infants sometimes tend to overrate the skills of their children. Some key clinical information about the child's motor development can be ascertained by asking them some broad open-ended questions[4] **(Table 1)**.

Children with increased tone may attain motor milestones which may be early, asymmetrical, or "out of order," like standing before sitting or development of handedness. If development of handedness is noticed before 18 months, you must look out for hemiparesis.

Children with CP may have associated problems, which may require diagnosis and referrals.

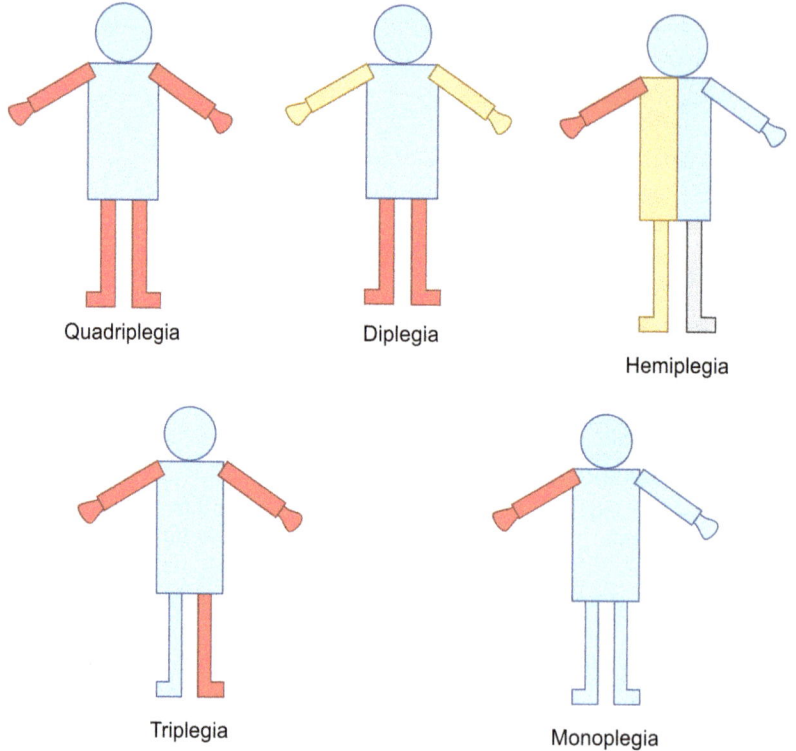

Fig. 3: Topographic classification of cerebral palsy.

TABLE 1: Key points in motor history.

Key Points	Example
Delayed acquisition of skill	Is there anything your child is not doing that you think he or she should be able to do?
Involuntary movements or coordination impairment	Is there anything your child is doing that you are concerned about?
Strength Coordination and endurance issues	Is there anything other children of the same age can do, that is difficult for your child?
Regression of skill	Is there any activity which your child was able to do which he or she cannot do now?

- *Cognitive problems*: The children may turn out to be underachievers in school, with delay in social and language problems. The delay may be due to associated sensory impairment.
- *Speech and language problems*: This may be due to hearing impairment or due to cognitive problems. Articulation defects may occur due to oromotor dysfunction.
- *Sensory impairment*: Hearing impairment, cortical blindness, and perceptual deficits
- *Ocular*: Strabismus, optic atrophy, and refractive errors
- *Seizures*: One-third of the patients may have seizures within the first 2 years, which are difficult to control and may need multiple anticonvulsants.

- *Gastrointestinal*: Constipation, gastroesophageal reflux disease (GERD), and poor dental hygiene
- *Nutrient deficiencies*: Poor exposure to sunlight, poor calcium intake, decreased intake of food, may all cause deficiency of vitamin D and micronutrients
- Pain may be due to muscle spasms, dental caries, constipation, or GERD. This may result in excessive crying and irritability.
- *Orthopedic*: Joint contractures, disparity in limb length due to spasticity, scoliosis of lumbar spine, hip subluxation, and talipes equinovarus are some of the complications. Low-impact fractures may occur due to osteopenia. All this may result in "crouch gait."
- Bladder problems

Modern neonatal intensive care has contributed to increased survival of infants at the limits of prematurity and to changes in the rates of neonatal morbidities and neurodevelopmental impairments. Recent studies suggest changes in both the rates of CP and the degree of severity. In the Neonatal Research Network Study,[5] extreme preterm infants born ≤27 weeks, were evaluated at 18–24 months. They showed that the rate of severe CP had decreased, but the rate of mild CP had increased. Although the incidence of major disability such as CP has decreased in extremely low birth weight (ELBW) infants, more subtle problems with motor coordination, executive function, and behavior were more frequent with decreasing gestation. They described a range of motor abnormalities including delayed motor milestones, balance abnormalities, challenges with manual dexterity, and generalized coordination abnormalities as Developmental Coordination Disorder (DCD), diagnosed with the Movement Assessment Battery (MABC-2).

Many preterm infants show abnormal signs in early infancy, which resolve by the age of 12 months and these are called "transient tone abnormalities."[6] Several abnormalities must be present and persist during sequential examinations before a diagnosis of CP is confirmed. Hence, a definitive diagnosis must not be made until the child is 12–18 months old.

In the Western world,[7] spastic CP is reported in 85% of cases. The PGIMER, Chandigarh, data reports 73% to be spastic CP (quadriplegia 51.5%, diplegic 34.5%, and hemiplegic 13.8%), 11.2% hypotonic/ataxic, and 8.8% mixed.[8]

Danger signals in preterm developmental patterns are shown in a tabular form to make it easy to use **(Table 2)**. The first column represents commonly seen behaviors in preterm infants. If several variables are present, and they persist, they could have a negative impact on the development of motor, sensory, and cognitive skills. The second column lists the interventions that can be done at home by parents. If several signs persist, referral to a therapist must be done. The third column lists the danger signals which are indications for referral to an occupational therapist. The fourth column shows the impact on later development due to this early deviant development and indicates why early referral is important.[10]

TABLE 2: Danger signs—preterm developmental patterns.

Preterm variables	Suggestions for Parents	Danger signals	Impact on later development
By 2 months (corrected age)			
Tone and Posture			
• Tendency to arch in extension • Legs extended instead of flexed posture • May have tremors of arms, legs, or chin • Hands may be intermittently fisted	• Position and carry the infant in flexed and midline postures	• Persistent arching in extension • Legs stiff/scissoring • Marked floppiness • Hands always fisted or no grasp elicited	• Delayed rolling, sitting, and crawling • Decreased ability to grasp and manipulate toys
Reflexes			
May have several beats of clonus		• Absence of primitive reflexes • Exaggerated startle • Sustained clonus	Clonus may interfere with standing and walking skills
Movement Skills			
May not be able to raise head above 30° when prone	• In prone, support under chest • Prop on caregiver's chest or hold upright at caregiver's shoulder	• Little or no active movement of arms and legs • Moves one side more than the other • Inability to hold head upright briefly (for 2 or 3 seconds) in pull to sit	Delayed gross motor skills
Behavior			
May have fewer or shorter quiet alert states than full-term infants	Provide dim lights and quiet environment to promote eye opening and visual attention	• Inability to respond to calming strategies, "difficult temperament," sensitive infant • Hypo- or hyperresponsive to environmental stimulation • Crying to loud or sudden sounds	Difficulty establishing self-regulatory strategies for sleep, attention, social interaction

Contd...

Contd...

Preterm variables	Suggestions for Parents	Danger signals	Impact on later development
Social Skills/Play			
Focuses only on face or toy in line of vision	• Encourage visual tracking by slowly moving toy or caregiver's face from midline to sides and vice versa	• Does not focus on face or toy	• Impact on development of social skills and learning
Feeding			
• May need encouragement to maintain an alert state to complete feedings • May need supplemental feedings due to poor oral motor skills	• Provide a quiet, calming environment for feedings • Establish a schedule for feedings, but respond to signs of hunger/demand behaviors	• Turns dusky, gags, or chokes with feedings • Feedings take longer than 40 minutes • May resist or refuse feedings	• At risk for aspiration • Work of feeding may exceed calorie intake and reduce weight gain
By 4 months (Corrected Age)			
Tone and Posture			
• Legs held mostly extended • Tendency to arch into an extended position in response to discomfort, excitment • Hands may be intermittently fisted, but open easily	• Position with legs in flexion and together (use towel or blanket rolls to assist) • Position frequently in side-lying for play • Massage hands open and bring open hands to knees, mouth, and toys	• Marked floppiness • Persistent arching in extension • Hands persistently fisted • Pull-to-sit results in infant pulling up to a stand	• Secondary deformities, especially of hips and spine • Inability to move against gravity • Inability to manipulate toys
Reflexes			
Neonatal positive support, palmar grasp, and moro may not be fully integrated, but infant can overcome them	Avoid standing or bouncing infant on feet	• *Presence of pathologic reflexes:* Sustained clonus, brisk deep tendon reflexes • Exaggerated startle to sound, visual stimuli, and/or movement	• Lack variety of movement skills • Inability to sustain movements and tasks

Contd...

Contd...

Preterm variables	Suggestions for Parents	Danger signals	Impact on later development
Movement Skills			
• May have difficulty moving against gravity (pushing up in prone) • Rolling front to back may not be controlled and may cause startle	• Towel rolls behind head and shoulders and under hip and knees in sit/supine to maintain a flexed position • Encourage bringing head and hands to midline	• More movement on one side versus the other, or arms versus legs • Strong resistance to prone; unable to lift head or persistent arching when prone • Unable to maintain head upright in sitting	• Asymmetry in movement and skill development • Delayed or poor-quality crawl/sit • Delayed walking
Behavior			
• Shorter, distinct quite alert times	• Reduce excessive noise, lights, and activity in environment	• Startles, jitters/tremors; cries frequently with movement, noise, or stimulation • Sleeps excessively	• Difficulty establishing self-regulatory strategies for sleep, attention, social interaction
Social Skills/Play			
• Excitement with person or toy results in extensor posturing • May not reach out for toys in supine position	• Dampen or limit extension by holding infant in flexion • Provide hand-overhand assistance and rattles that fasten with velcro around wrists	• Does not smile with friendly interactions • Shows little interest or does not attempt to track a toy or face • Does not bring hands to mouth	• Poor development of social interaction • Reduced opportunity for hand exploration and use of hands for self-calming
Feeding			
• May be unable to feed well in a new or highly stimulating environment	• Avoid feeding in new or highly stimulating environments	• Coughs, chokes, or gags frequently • Resists or refuses feedings • Arches and cries during or after feedings	• Poor growth • At risk for aspiration • Poor development of feeding skills
By 6 months (Corrected Age)			
Tone and Posture			
• May continue to have mild stiffness or floppiness • May continue to dislike and avoid prone	• Continue to encourage proper positioning in prone • Discourage standing and use of walkers if showing fixing patterns	• Asymmetries predominate • In supported sit—back-rounded and frog-legged position, or baby pushes back with legs stiff and feet plantar—flexed	• Development of skeletal deformities • Inability to free hands for play • Difficulty crawling • Difficulty with standing and walking independently

Contd...

Cerebral Palsy

Contd...

Preterm variables	Suggestions for Parents	Danger signals	Impact on later development
		• Stands on toes with stiff legs or with wide base, or will not bear weight on legs • Difficulty opening hands and reaching for objects in any position	
Reflexes			
• May move in and out of reflexive postures	• Encourage a variety of positions and vary methods of carrying and holding	• Strong, persistent primitive reflexes that may affect movement patterns (e.g., ATNR, moro)	• Problems with independent sitting, increased probability of deformities
Movement Skills			
• May not be able to shift weight well in prone to reach for a toy	• Position so infant can kick suspended toys • Use colorful socks on feet • In prone, position toys to sides instead of centered in front of the infant	• Unable to bear weight on hands or forearms in prone or sit • Rolling in one direction only • Head lag in pull-to-sit	• Poor development of shoulder girdle/muscles affecting upper extremity • Progress in gross motor skill development impaired
Behavior			
• May have only one successful method of self-calming	• Provide organization strategies (such as use of music, or favorite toy) to assist with transitions	• Overwhelmed by sensory demands of interactions of handling (bathing, diaper changes) • Persistent startle to sounds and movement change	• Negative impact on daily routines
Social Skills/Play			
• Shakes, bangs, and explores toys, but may lack control • Attention span for social interaction and play may be brief	• Limit the number of toys provided at one time; be conscious of overstimulation	• Difficulty opening hands and reaching for objects in any position • Does not explore hands or toys with mouth • Does not make cooing or babbling sounds	• Potential for contractures and lack of fine motor skills • Impaired development of social interactions

Contd...

Contd...

Preterm variables	Suggestions for Parents	Danger signals	Impact on later development
Feeding			
• May lose pureed food from mouth due to tongue protrusion pattern	• Practice spoon feeding without worrying about volume of intake	• Refuses spoon feedings • Strong tongue thrusting results in large volume loss from mouth • Coughs, chokes, or gags frequently with feedings	• Failure to thrive • Poor development of feeding skills • At risk for aspiration
By 9 months (Corrected Age)			
Tone and Posture			
• May prefer extended postures, (e.g., standing as opposed to sitting) • Frequently stands on toes, but can come down to flat feet • Feet may be pronated, and knees locked in standing if mildly hypotonic	• Sit, with support if necessary, and play with toys at feet • Discourage standing, use of walkers	• Strong arching • Stands on toes consistently, with legs stiff. May have scissoring of legs • Unable to bear weight on legs in supported stand	Difficulty sitting independently Transition to walking impaired
Reflexes			
• May continue to see subtle influences of ATNR	• Position head in midline in pram	• Pathologic reflexes present (e.g., positive Babinski, clonus, hyperreflexive tendon reflexes)	• Poor development of reciprocal patterns for walking and crawling
Movement Skills			
• Creeps, no crawl • May not be able to assume or maintain a sitting position	• In sitting, position toys off to the side, slightly out of reach • Work on crawling	• Unable to sit and prop forward independently or sit with hands free to play	• Difficulty with crawling • Secondary deformities
Behavior			
• May be overwhelmed more frequently in new or noisy environments	• Be aware of environmental factors and their impact on child	• Parents describe infant as wide-eyed, hyper, or easily overstimulated	• Compromised attention and potential for learning

Contd...

Contd...

Preterm variables	Suggestions for parents	Danger signals	Impact on later development
Social Skills/Play			
• Able to pick up small objects, but with immature grasp	• Hand child small objects rather than have him/her pick them up from a surface	• Does not show interest in or explore toys with hands or mouth • Does not initiate simple gestures, play or sounds	• Poor development of tool use (e.g., pencils spoons) • Limitations in cognitive development
Feeding			
• May have difficulty progressing in diet (e.g., to solids, new foods)	• Offer foods at least three times per day, providing a variety of tastes and textures	• Gags on or refuses solid foods	• Inability to transition to table foods
By 12 months (Corrected Age)			
Tone and Posture			
• May prefer "W" sitting • Mild foot pronation when standing	• Encourage a variety of sitting patterns • Shoes with good arches give more support and may decrease toe-standing	• Only able to "W" sit; unable to maintain sitting in other positions • Stands on toes with legs stiff and adducted	• Joint and bony deformities • Poor play skills • Difficulty transitioning to independent walking
Reflexes			
• Reflexes are integrated; may see influence only under stress		• Retention of any developmental or pathologic reflexes	• Unable to develop higher-level motor skills
Movement Skills			
• May still have a wide base when walking	• Practice walking with one hand-held	• Not getting into sitting position or up on hands and knees independently • Not crawling on hands and knees; may bunny-hop • Not pulling to stand • Not cruising	• Delayed motor skills
Behavior			
• May display short attention span and be easily distracted	• Continue to modify the environment to minimize distractions	• Daily care is consistently difficult (e.g., bathing, dressing, and feeding)	

Contd...

Contd...

Preterm variables	Suggestions for parents	Danger signals	Impact on later development
Social Skills/Play			
• May require child to imitate caregiver to fully explore toys	• Encourage engagement in one aspect of toy, then add additional sensory components	• Does not imitate simple sounds or gestures • Does not follow simple verbal requests • Excessive mouthing of toys or persistent lack of oral exploration	• Delayed language skills • Limited cognitive development
Feeding			
• May not yet have transitioned from bottle or breast to cup	• Provide many opportunities to practice drinking from a cup, offering a variety of beverages	• Consistently gags, cries, and resists feedings • Strong tongue thrusting pattern with spoon feedings	• Child may acquire maladaptive eating skills and develop strong food refusal behaviors

(ATNR: asymmetrical tonic neck reflex)

TABLE 3: Topography and magnetic resonance imaging (MRI) findings.

Topographic classification	MRI findings
Quadriplegic CP	Periventricular white matter changes in the form of cysts/leukomalacia with changes of volume loss
Diplegic CP	Cortical/subcortical lesions such as encephalomalacic changes, cortical dysplasia, and polymicrogyria
Hemiplegic CP	Unilateral lesions, bilateral (more extensive on one side), focal lesions such as cortical/subcortical insults, and cortical malformations
Dyskinetic CP	• Basal ganglia lesions • Deep nuclei lesions/scars, hippocampal lesions

(CP: cerebral palsy)

After the diagnosis is confirmed and explained to the parents, they are completely flustered and want to know "why" this happened to their child. A magnetic resonance imaging (MRI) of the brain at this stage may help. One can point out the lesion to them and explain the damage done to a certain part of the brain **(Table 3)**. At the same time, one must explain the concept of "plasticity" of the brain and why early intervention is important and encourage them to remain positive.

Before starting therapy, the Gross Motor Function Classification (GMFCS-B and E) may be used to categorize the patient.

TABLE 4: Drugs used to reduce spasticity.

Indication	Drug	Mechanism of action	Dose	Side effects
Generalized spasticity	Baclofen	GABA-B agonist	0.2–2 mg/kg/day BD/TDS oral	Headache, seizures, urinary retention, insomnia
	Diazepam	Facilitates GABA-A receptor-mediated presynaptic inhibition	0.5–0.75 BD oral	Sedation, tolerance, withdrawal seizures
	Tizanidine	Central α-2 noradrenergic agonist	0.3–05 mg/kg/day QID oral	Dry mouth, somnolence, dizziness, asthenia
	Dantrolene	Muscle relaxant	0.5–10 mg/kg/day BD oral	Sedation, CNS effects, GIT effects
Localized spasticity	Botulinum A toxin	Prevents presynaptic release of acetylcholine at neuromuscular junction	• Large muscle 4–6 u/kg • Small muscle 1–2 u/kg • Limited to maximum 400–600 u IM	Unwanted paralysis of adjacent muscles, pain, rash, malaise

(CNS: central nervous system; GABA: gamma-aminobutyric acid; GIT: gastrointestinal tract)

IMPORTANCE OF EARLY INTERVENTION

Intervention is most important in CP for the following reasons:
- For infants having the potential to have normal movement patterns, therapy helps to build a foundation on which future movement skills can be built. The main aim is inhibition of abnormal movement patterns.[9]
- The development of normal movements at the appropriate age allows the infant to experience more normal vestibular and sensorimotor stimulation.
- The success of neurodevelopmental therapy depends on the therapist's ability to make changes in muscle tone.
- The help of certain drugs such as baclofen may be taken to reduce spasticity. This reduces the difficulty for the therapist and the parents who carry out the exercises at home **(Table 4)**.
- For those infants, who may never have normal tone, the therapist can teach them certain functional patterns which require less energy and prevent orthopedic deformities. Parents can be taught proper handling techniques to maximize their child's skills. For instance, oil massage should not be done in children who have had seizures and are discharged home on Gardenal, as this may stimulate spasms of hypertonia.
- Family members can be counseled how best to help the child, especially those children who will have permanent neurologic deficit. The parents need a lot of moral support from the therapist and doctor, not only to accept the diagnosis, but also to cope with this situation.

- The main aim of therapy is to prevent contractures, muscle imbalance resulting in deformities such as scoliosis, hip dislocation, foot positioning problems, excessive drooling and feeding problems leading to aspiration **(Table 4)**.

It is important to give dietary advice. In young children, calorie-dense balanced diet must be advised. However, in older nonambulatory children, calories should be cut down to prevent obesity, especially during adolescence. Parents should be alerted regarding sexual abuse in girls. School placement is a major problem in India. Children with CP with normal intellect can attend regular school, but absence of ramps in school causes great difficulty. Those with borderline intelligence may need special education, if they cannot be managed with integrated schooling. The children may also develop many emotional problems, since they are different from normal children.

Parents need a lot of emotional support and should be encouraged to form Parent Support Groups. Mothers should be counseled that they should not be obsessed with this "special" child, but spare enough time for the rest of the family.

REFERENCES

1. Surveillance of Cerebral Palsy in Europe. A collaboration of cerebral palsy surveys and registers. Dev Med Child Neurol. 2000;42(12):816-24.
2. Chauhan A, Singh M, Jaiswal N, Agarwal A, Sahu JK, Singh M. Prevalence of cerebral palsy in Indian children: a systematic review and meta-analysis. Ind J Pediatr. 2018;86(12):1124-30.
3. Chaudhari S, Kulkarni S, Barve S, Pandit A, Sonak U, Sarpotdar N. Neurologic sequelae in high-risk infants: a three-year follow up. Indian Pediatr. 1996;33(8):645-53.
4. Novitz GH, Murphy NA and Neuromotor Screening Panel. Pediatrics. 2013;131e:2016.
5. McGowan EC, Vohr BR. Neurodevelopmental follow up of preterm infants: what is new? Pediatr Clin North Am. 2019;66(2):509-23.
6. Tagare A, Chaudhari S, Kadam S, Vaidya UV, Pandit A, Sayyad MG. Mortality and morbidity in extremely low birth (ELBW) infants in neonatal intensive care unit. Indian J Pediatr. 2013;80(1):16-20.
7. Rosenbaum P, Paneth N, Leviton A, Goldstein M, Bax M, Damiano D, et al. A report: definition and classification of cerebral palsy. Dev Med Child Neurol Suppl. 2007;109: 8-14.
8. Singhi P, Saini AG. Changes in clinical spectrum of cerebral palsy over two decades in North India: an analysis of 1212 cases of cerebral palsy. J Trop Pediatr. 2013;59(6):434-40.
9. Berbaum J. Hoffman-Williamson M. Primary care of the preterm infant. Philadelphia: Mosby Yearbook; 1991. pp. 240-9.

CHAPTER 8A

Early Intervention

Sudha Chaudhari

INTRODUCTION

The brain is an incredibly complex structure. The development of the brain begins with the formation of the neural plate. Neurogenesis starts at 5 weeks gestational age and peaks at 25 weeks. The development of the brain occurs in an orderly fashion. Neurogenesis is followed by neuronal proliferation, migration, and aggregation. Then, axonal growth and formation of synapses occur. Synaptogenesis and migration proceed at a rapid rate till the end of the third year. Then, this process slows down and continues at a reduced rate.[1]

The brain has tremendous plasticity. The word plasticity is derived from the Greek word "plasticos," which means to form. This refers to the flexibility of the brain and its ability to adapt and change according to experience. Neural plasticity, the ability of the brain to be shaped by good or bad experiences, is at its peak during the "critical period." The neurons or synapses which are activated repeatedly are preserved and those which are not used, are pruned. Thus, the brain has enhanced plasticity during early childhood.[2] There is persistence of neurogenesis in certain parts of the brain in the postnatal period. Deletion of neurons through apoptosis or programmed cell death, proliferation and pruning of synapses, and activity-dependent refinement of synaptic connections occur during the first 3 years of life **(Fig. 1)**. Total brain

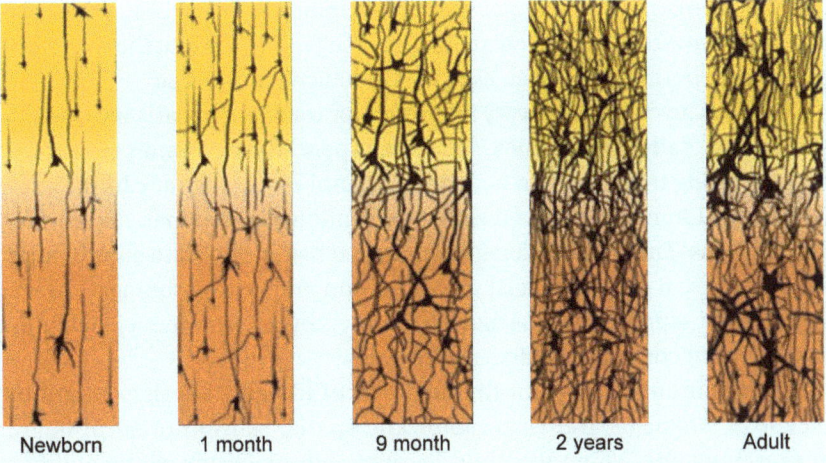

Fig. 1: Synaptic connections at different ages.

volume doubles in the first year of life and is 83% of the adult volume by the end of 2 years. The cerebellum also shows dramatic changes during this period. The first 3 years of life is a critical period during which our experiences have its peak effect on development, normal behavior, and learning. The double neocortical circuitry, in which the subplate and cortical plate circuitries coexist, is gradually replaced by a single circuitries of the development network in the cortical plate. Early intervention will have its maximum effect during this period, which is the first three years of life.[3] The sensory experiences, stimulation, and language stimulation during this period may determine myelination and neuronal connectivity. The principle "use it or lose it" and "use it and grow it" applies to plasticity of the brain.

Early intervention services are meant for children who are at risk for developing delay or those who already have established delay in the age group of birth to 3 years. A child is considered to have developmental delay, if there is a delay in one or more of the following areas:
- Physical development—including fine or gross motor function
- Cognitive development
- Communication development
- Social and emotional development
- Adaptive development

The delay may be due to neurologic diseases, genetic problems, or visual and hearing impairment. The group that benefits the most is the high-risk babies discharged from the neonatal intensive care unit (NICU).

Delayed motor, cognitive, and emotional impairment due to biologic or environmental risk factors will be prevented or minimized by early intervention. The amazingly improved intellectual performance of an orphan child, adopted into a caring and stimulating home, is a classic example of environmental intervention. It was believed that this did not hold true for a child with brain injury as neurons are not "regenerable." However, animal studies in neurophysiology have shown that synapses are regenerable, if not neurons. The concept of synapse sculpturing indicates that neurotransmission can be improved by selectively stabilizing one type of insult at the expense of others[4] and both these processes can be enhanced by training.[5]

Parental involvement is very important for transferring early intervention practices in daily life activities, since they spend the maximum time caring and nurturing the child.[6,7] In a study by Gianni et al.,[8] very low birth weight (VLBW) children who received early intervention were compared to controls at 36 months. The intervention group showed better eye–hand coordination, higher scores in personal social subscales, and practical reasoning. However, some recent reports have questioned whether this improvement in cognitive development continues in later school years.[9]

Intervention provided in the first year of life may advance cognition, receptive language, and visuomotor and spatial skills in preterm infants at preschool age. When the child learns to sit, he improves the ability to process visual information. Cognitive development in the future is facilitated

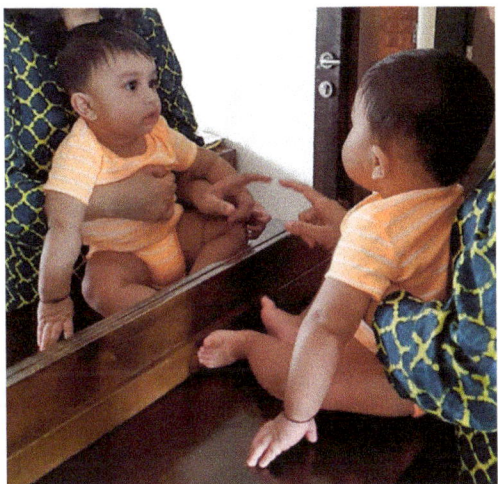

Fig. 2: To encourage eye-hand coordination and to learn body parts.

by the interaction of postural control and visual attention. Visual attention is a key factor in problem-solving **(Fig. 2)**. The coordination of improved gaze stabilization and manual skills during sitting is accompanied by object interaction and learning. Sitting allows infants to use their hands freely to put objects and take them apart, a behavior that forms the foundation for understanding mathematical concepts.

Cognitive development in the initial stages is interdependent on the sensory systems—vision, hearing, tactile, vestibular and proprioceptive, and also the motor area. At 6-7 months, most infants can sit. This would not have been possible if the infant had not developed head control against gravity and extension of the spine. The motor development proceeds in a cephalocaudal and proximal to distal fashion. The inter-relationships between their bodies, objects, and people, are understood by the infant by sitting, objective interaction and locomotion activities and this in turn enhances their cognition.[10] These behaviors are complex, dynamic, and evolving throughout the first year of life. Normal infants perform these behaviors sequentially during the first year. Although developmental trajectories may differ, the sequence always remains the same.

The intervention may include occupational or physical therapy, speech therapy, therapy for visual problems, and other services based on the needs of the child.[11] This will have a significant impact on the child's ability to learn new skills and increase their success in school life. The neural circuits in the brain, which are the foundation for learning, behavior, and health, are the most adaptable in the first 3 years of life. They will become harder to change afterward.

So, the goals of early intervention are:
- Acceleration of the rate of development in the child
- Acquisition of new behaviors and skills by the child
- Increase in independent functioning

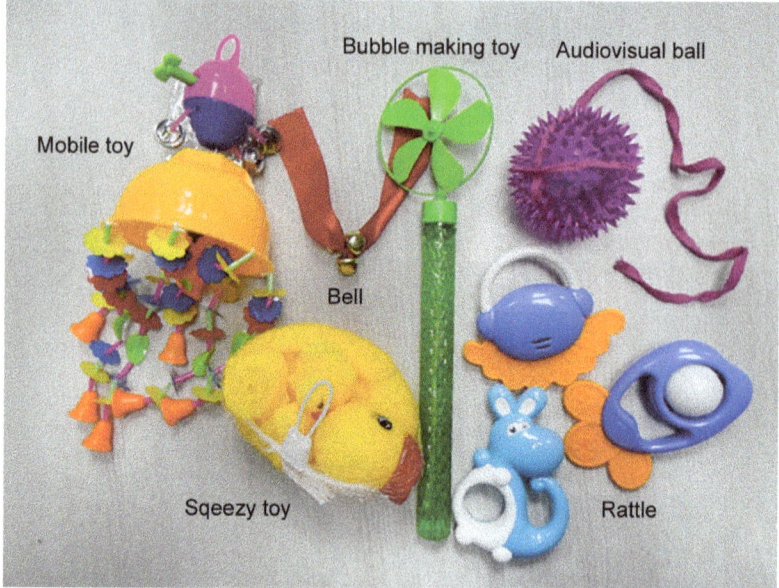

Fig. 3: Stimulation kit.

- Minimization of the effects of handicapping conditions
- Early detection and prevention of secondary handicaps
- To render assistance to parents in coping skills and understanding their child's development

At the KEM Hospital, Pune, we conduct three "High Risk Clinics" per week, where NICU graduates are followed up regularly. A detailed developmental assessment is done by the occupational therapist at 3, 6, 9, and 12 months and a developmental quotient (DQ) is done at 18 months. Corrected age is used in preterm infants. If any delay is noticed, the mother is advised a stimulation program at home. A special stimulation kit **(Fig. 3)** is given free of charge along with an instruction sheet **(Annexure IV)**. If the baby shows severe delay, then the baby is referred to the in-house TDH Rehabilitation Centre and Morris Child Development Centre for further therapy. It is important to start the therapy as early as possible for a good outcome.

REFERENCES

1. Gioranni C, Inguaggiato E, Sgandurra G. Early intervention in neurodevelopmental disorders: underlying neural mechanism. Dev Med Child Neurol. 2016;58(Suppl 4):61-8.
2. Mundkur N. Neuroplasticity in children. Ind J Pediatr. 2005;72(10):855-7.
3. Noyes-Grosser D, Holland J, Lyons D, Holland C, Romanczyk R, Gillis J. Rationale and methodology for developing guidelines for early intervention services for young children with developmental disabilities. Infants Young Child. 2005;18(2):119-35.
4. Simecosson RJ, Cooper DH, Schneir AP. A review and analysis of the effectiveness of early intervention program. Pediatrics. 1982;69(5):635-41.
5. Report of the Panel of Developmental Neurologic Disorders to the NANC Stroke Council Public No.(NIH);1979. pp. 18-74.

6. Guralnick MJ. Why early intervention works? Infant Young Child. 2011;24(1):6-28.
7. Hadders-Algra M. Early diagnosis and early intervention. Front Neurol. 2014;6:185.
8. Gianni ML, Picciolini O, Ravasi M, Gardon L, Vegni C, Fumagalli M, et al. The effects of early developmental mother-child intervention program on neurodevelopmental outcome in very low birth weight infants. Early Hum Dev. 2006;82(10):691-5.
9. McGowan EC, Vohr BR. Neurodevelopmental follow up of preterm infants. What is new? Pediatr Clin North Am. 2019;66(2):509-23.
10. Bonnier C. Evaluation of early stimulation programs for enhancing brain development. Acta Pediatr. 2008;97(7):853-58.
11. Johnston MV. Clinical disorders of brain plasticity. Brain Dev. 2004;26(2):73-80.

CHAPTER 8B

Occupational Therapy with Emphasis on a Home-based Stimulation Program

Bharati Patil

INTRODUCTION

The aim of occupational therapy and physiotherapy is to bridge the gap between impaired development and normalcy. Therapy is based on inhibition of abnormal reflex movement patterns and facilitation of normal development. The goals are normal motor development, which includes normalization of tone, improving joint range of motion, and improving posture and balance reactions.

The therapist evaluates the baby by a physical examination, which includes tone, voluntary control, mode of locomotion, reflex activity, and hand function. She also observes carrying pattern, posture, and movement pattern. Special attention is given to the difficulties in activities of daily living (ADL) such as feeding, dressing, and toilet care.

Therapeutic exercises are planned as per each child's requirement and the frequency of visits to the center is also decided. The mother is by the side of the baby 24 × 7 and is the best person who can provide therapy and stimulation at home. This not only improves parent–child bonding, but also reduces stress and gives them the satisfaction of doing something and contributing to the child's development. The aim of therapy is to develop gross and fine motor skills required to gain independence in ADL, along with perceptual and cognitive development.

All infants discharged from the neonatal intensive care unit are followed up in the High-risk Clinic. At the KEM Hospital, Pune, the clinic is held three times a week and an occupational therapist regularly attends the clinic. A neurodevelopmental assessment is done by her using our own assessment method at 3, 6, 9, and 12 months (**Annexure III**). If any delay is suspected, a home-based stimulation program is given to the parents, along with a free stimulation kit (*See* **Chapter 8A**). They are called to the clinic after a month, and if the delay persists, they are referred to the in-house TDH Rehabilitation Centre for therapy (**Fig. 1**).

At the center, a detailed history is taken. The type of family (joint or nuclear), nature of the job if both parents are working, number of siblings etc., is noted. The neurodevelopmental approach described by Bobath is used for assessment and therapy. The main principle of this therapy is inhibition of abnormal movement patterns and persistent neonatal reflexes and facilitation of normal development. Corrected age is used in preterm infants for assessment. Neurodevelopmental assessment is done in the following manner.

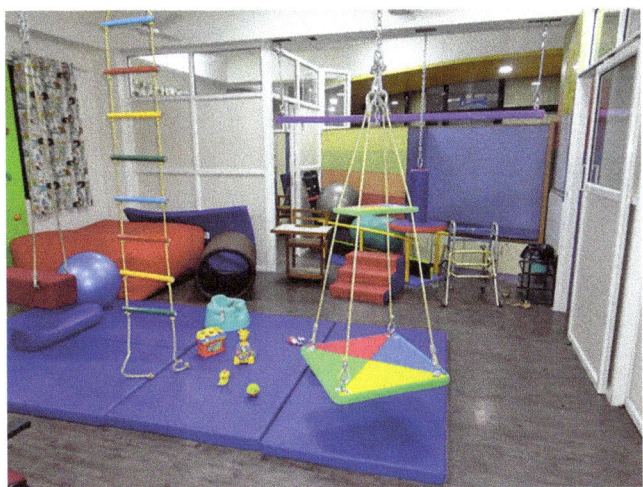

Fig. 1: Developmental therapy unit.

- The tone of the whole body is assessed:[1]
  - Hypertonia, hypotonia, or mixed tone
  - The milestones are noted.
  - Head control
  - Sitting with or without support, creeping, crawling, standing with or without support, walking with or without support
- The quality of the movement is assessed as per the following points:[2]
  - Full joint range of motion
  - Elongation of muscles
  - Weight bearing on proximal joints
  - Weight shifts, anterior, posterior, and lateral
  - Vision is assessed by visual contact and pursuit and other visual problems such as nystagmus and squint are noted.
  - For hearing assessment, babbling is present or absent, the overall interaction of the child with parents and surrounding people, is also noted.

After the neurodevelopmental assessment, problems of ADL such as feeding and dressing, depending on the age of the child, are evaluated. The parents are extremely anxious when they are referred to the rehabilitation center. So, the first duty of the therapist is to reassure the parents and point out the positive points in the development of their child. For instance, it can be pointed out that the mental development of the child looks good and this can be a reassuring point. A detailed discussion of the plus points as well as the delayed issues should be done and parents are encouraged to have a positive attitude. In a joint family, counseling of the whole family may be necessary, especially the mother-in-law, who is a very important person in our social and cultural system. When the new parents are waiting for a therapy session, other parents who have been coming for some time, also talk to them and encourage them.

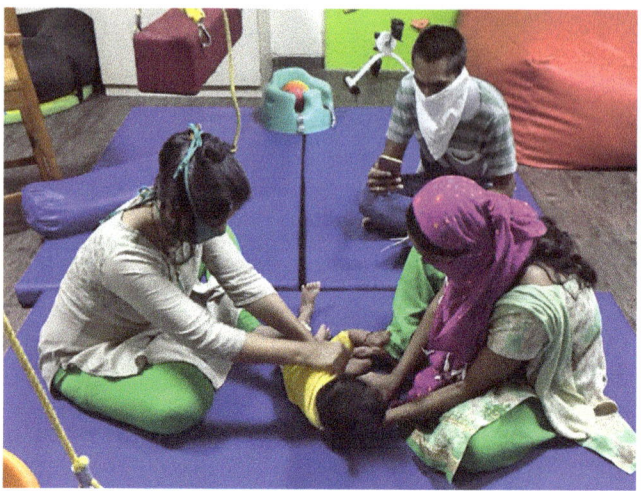

Fig. 2: Father taking video.

THERAPY PLAN

Short-term and long-term goals should be set. The short-term goals for 0–3 months are proper positioning while feeding, dressing, and carrying, active neck control on prone position and inhibition of persistent neonatal reflexes, and normalization of tone. The long-term goal will be walking by 2 years. When the therapist is teaching the exercises to the mother, the father is asked to shoot a video so that the mother can do the exercises at home more confidently **(Fig. 2)**.

TECHNIQUES FOR NORMALIZING TONE

- *Hypertonia*: Reduce the tone by gentle stretching by passive range of motion and myofascial release. Massage should be avoided.
- *Hypotonia*: Improve tone by tapping and compressions
- *Mixed tone or fluctuating tone*: Facilitate controlled coordinated movements

HOME-BASED STIMULATION PROGRAM

Tummy Time

At 3–4 months, the baby should be placed in the prone position at least 4–5 times a day, when awake. The prone position facilitates extension against gravity, shoulder girdle stability, which is most important for gaining neck control and development of fine motor skills. It also enhances anteroposterior weight shifts for developing trunk extensors. It inhibits asymmetrical tonic neck reflex (ATNR) and tonic labyrinthine reflex and extensor hypertonus.

Head Control (3–4 Months)[3]

- To raise the head, place the child in the prone position with elbows under the shoulders. Hold the shoulders and pull them toward the spine.

When the child lifts the head, show a bright colored toy and move it up and down. Once the child holds the head, move the toy sideways.
- Place the child in the mother's lap in the prone position. Stroke the neck muscles. Tap the forehead to encourage lifting the head.
- Carry the child in the prone position.
- Place the child on the mother's chest and talk to the child.
- Place the child in the prone position, and ask the mother to place a bright colored noise-making toy out of reach of the child and stimulate the child to move by holding one elbow under the shoulder. After placing the child in the prone position with one elbow under the shoulder, flex hip and knee on the same side, while applying a little pressure on the sole, so that child tries to creep.

Sitting with Support (5–6 Months)[4]

Supported sitting facilitates strengthening of back extensors as well as co-contraction between flexors of the trunk and extensors, for a stable trunk. Sitting expands the visual field and helps the child to reach forward.
- Make the child sit in the lap, supporting the trunk.
- Place the child in a Bumbo chair **(Fig. 3)**.
- Make the child sit in a corner of the room. Put a bolster in front and cushions at the back.
- To develop sitting balance, make the child sit on a big gym ball and move the ball in various directions. To improve trunk balance, let the child sit on the gym ball and reach for a toy **(Fig. 4)**.

Sitting without Support (7–9 Months)[5]

It is a very stable position. The hands get free for exploration and manipulation. Parachute reaction, backward and sideways, is developed. Can transition from crawl to sit and sit to crawl.

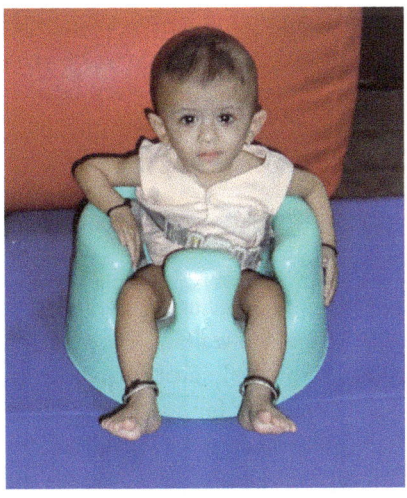

Fig. 3: Bumbo® chair.

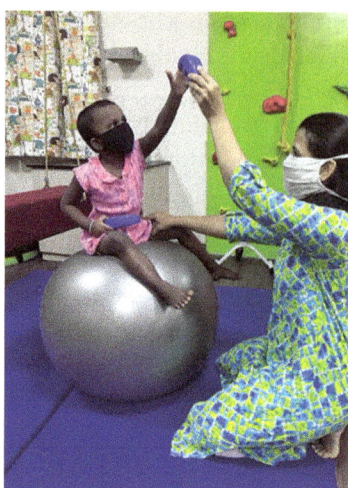

Fig. 4: Reaching out for a toy sitting on a gymnasium ball.

- Make the child sit on the floor with hands on the ground. Hold at the shoulder or pelvis, if required.
- Make the child sit cross-legged with one hand flat on the ground. Offer a toy in front of the other hand.
- Make the child sit with one leg flexed and the other leg extended, putting the hand flat on the ground, on the flexed leg side. Offer a toy on the same side. The child will turn by rotating the trunk and take the toy with the free hand.
- Make the child sit on a bolster with legs flat on the ground and play with the child in this position.
- Make the child sit on a ball and tilt it from side to side and back and front to improve balance.
- Make the child sit in a side-sitting position and encourage the child to go on all fours.
- Make the child sit in your lap and bounce the child.
- Make the child sit in your lap, hold both the legs at the knees, and move the child forward and backward to encourage weight bearing on legs.
- Let the child be in the supine position. Hold one shoulder and turn the child to the opposite side, while stabilizing the pelvis. Let the child come to sitting position by bearing weight on the elbows and hands.
- Avoid "W" sitting.

Crawling (8–11 Months)[4]

It is the most important milestone because it facilitates alternating pattern of hand and leg, which will be used in walking. It also gives shoulder girdle and pelvic girdle stability. Pressure on the heel of the palm during crawling develops palmar arches, which are important for fine motor development.

- Place the child in a crawling position on a small ball holding elbows straight and hands flat, with hips and knees flexed. Move forward and backward **(Fig. 5)**.

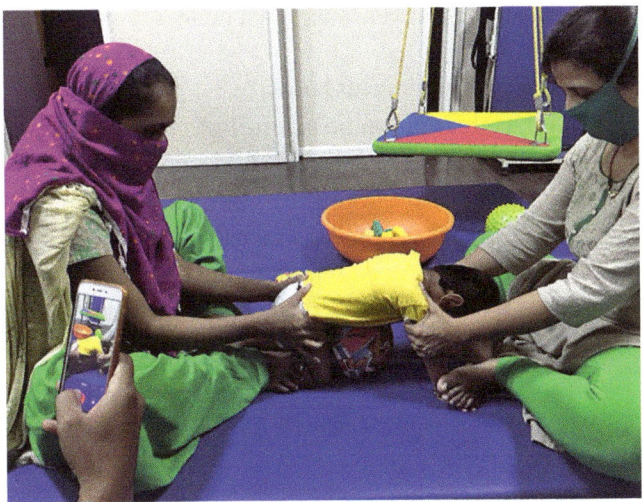

Fig. 5: Anterior-posterior weight shifts with a small ball in crawling position.

- Leave the child in a crawling position, let the child balance on all fours in this position and try to come up on the hands.
- Put the child in prone position, flex hips and knees, immobilize pelvis by holding it. Let the child come up using both the hands.
- Place the child in a crawling position. Offer a toy above one shoulder, so that he/she has to turn from the trunk to reach for the toy.
- Once the child attains the crawling position, hold the child by the elbows and knees and move them alternately. Two people are needed for this exercise.

Standing in a Kneeling Position (8–11 Months)[5]

The child can pull up to a kneeling position from a crawling position. This position is very important for trunk control and pelvic girdle stability.
- Encourage the child to hold on to furniture and pull up to kneeling position.
- Put the child in a kneeling position against a sofa, and put toys on the sofa. Let the child play with the toys in this position.
- Place the child in front of the mirror.
- Encourage the child to walk on both the knees.

Standing (11–13 Months)[4]

- Make the child sit in your lap with feet flat on the ground. Another person holds the knees from the front and pulls the knees in front. The person at the back supports the trunk. The child will pull up for standing.
- Make the child sit on a small table against the wall. Hold both the knees and pull them in front, the child will come to stand.
- Let the child hold on to window bars and pull up to stand.
- Make the child play in a squatting position. Move the child backward and forward.

- Make the child stand against a wall, put a table in front and let the child play **(Figs. 6 and 7)**.
- Make the child stand, holding his knees.
- Lift one leg, and let the child stand on one leg.
- Hold the child by the pelvis, and let the child walk.
- Posterior walker or pediatric walker can be used for supported walking. The usual popular walkers should not be used **(Fig. 8)**.
- Wrap a long cloth like a "dupatta" around the trunk. Hold both the ends from behind and let the child walk toward the mother, who is standing in front **(Fig. 9)**.

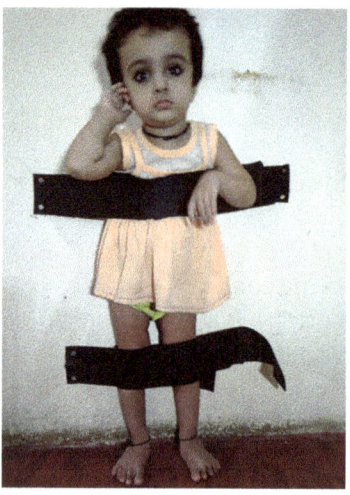

Fig. 6: Supported standing against wall.

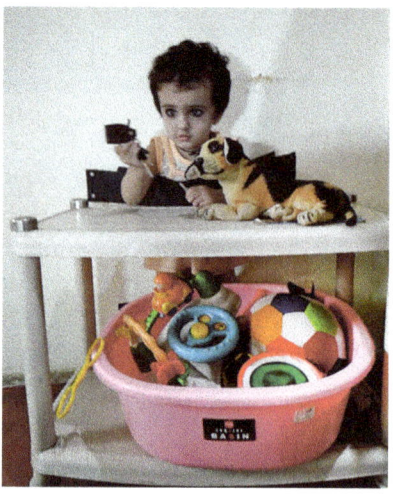

Fig. 7: Supported standing with a table full of toys in front.

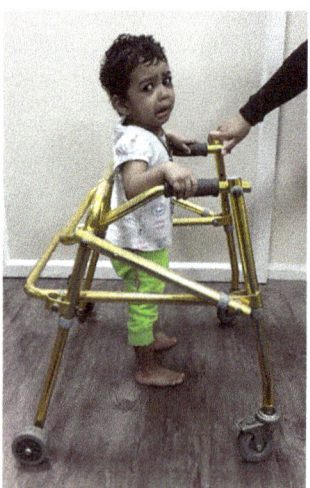

Fig. 8: Walking with a posterior walker.

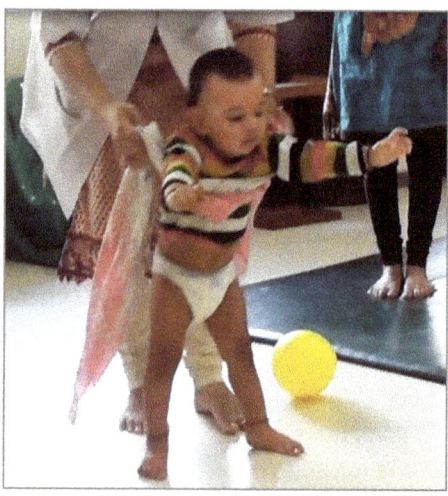

Fig. 9: Supported walking.

Even if the child is lagging behind in motor development, we encourage standing with proper support by 12–14 months. This gives the child the experience of weight-bearing on the lower limbs and holding the upright position. Children with hamstring tightness are advised a knee-ankle foot orthosis (KAFO), a splint from mid-thigh to foot or an ankle foot orthosis (AFO) which is a much lower splint. For babies with hypotonia and a flat foot, valgus insole is advised. The child should be made to stand at least 4–5 times a day.

There are some movements which are very difficult for a particular child.[6] For instance, the child with spastic quadriplegia finds it very difficult to come to a sitting or standing position. A child with diplegia finds it very difficult to crawl and usually has "bunny hopping." Half kneeling is very difficult for the child and the child will walk with a scissoring gait. A child with hemiplegia finds it difficult to crawl, has difficulty in bilateral activities, and fine motor activities. Most children with athetosis have nystagmus, and their fine motor activities are affected. They may walk with crutches or a walker. Monoplegia is usually a mild hemiplegia, and gross motor activities are affected due to balance issues.

DEVELOPMENT OF HAND FUNCTION

The child starts walking by 15–18 months and the hands become free from the task of uprighting. Hand function or fine motor coordination begins at 2 months when the infant starts bearing weight on forearms and gets refined, till the age of 6 years, when the child begins to write.

Stimulation (3–6 Months)

By the age of 3 months, the infant develops hand regard, tries to reach and claps hands together.

- Place the child in your lap in a semi-reclining position. Hold both the hands and let the child touch both cheeks.[5]
- Rub both hands with each other.
- Put the baby on the tummy and put a bright-colored toy in front of the child. Let the baby reach for it.
- Give a soft toy to hold, give a rattle.
- Make the baby sit in the lap and give a red ball to throw with both hands.
- Offer a toy on the opposite side, so that the baby turns and takes the toy, crossing the midline.
- Place the infant in a baby gym **(Fig. 10)**.
- Tie wrist bands, so that the baby is attracted to them.
- Massage fingers and toes. This is a very pleasurable activity for the baby and provides tactile sensory output.

Stimulation (6–9 Months)

- Allow the child to hold the bottle[7]
- Let the child bang noise-making toys
- Make the child sit in a high chair, and put toys in front on the tray

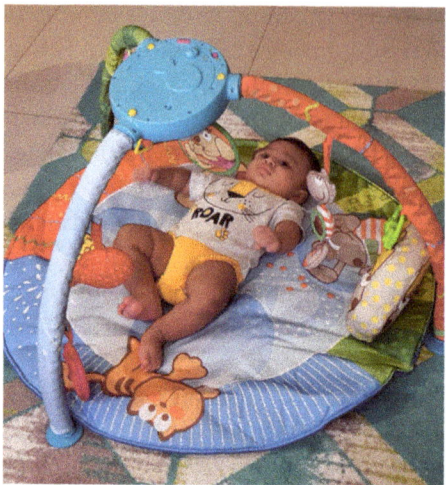

Fig. 10: Baby gymnasium.

- Show a book with colorful pictures and thick pages
- Let the child poke fingers in play dough
- Use peg boards and ring stands
- Put small finger foods such as raisins, sweet corn, puffed rice, in front of the child, and encourage the child to pick it up and eat.

Stimulation (10–12 Months)

- Give big size beads to pick up
- Give a book with thick pages and teach the child how to turn pages
- Give the child blocks and teach the child to stack them one on top of another
- Putting and taking out pegs from a peg board
- Small pieces of food to pick-up and eat
- Thick crayons to scribble
- Place a spoon in the hand of the baby and take it to the mouth.

While doing all these activities, the mother should be continuously talking to the child.

Activities of Daily Living

Activities of daily living such as dressing, undressing, bathing, toilet care, and feeding, are routine for normal children. But these are difficult in children with tone abnormalities and mothers are counseled on how to do these routine activities in these "special" children.

Carrying Patterns[4]

- Carrying a child with extensor spasticity. Flex the child by the shoulder girdle and turn the child to the side. Pick-up the child from the front and hold the child in a flexed position **(Fig. 11)**.
- A child who has good neck and trunk control can be carried at the waist.

Occupational Therapy with Emphasis on a Home-based Stimulation Program

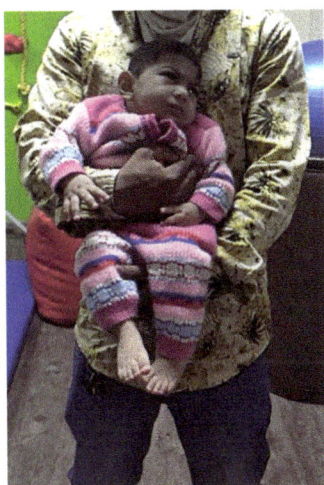

Fig. 11: Carrying position for a child with extensor hypertonia.

- Carrying a child with flexor spasticity and is curled up—arms should be elevated above the shoulders, with head held up. Stretch the trunk, support pelvic region, and let the legs hang.
- Carrying a child with athetosis or a floppy child. The child is carried in the same way as a child with extensor spasticity.

Control of Drooling

Make the child sit in a reclining position in your lap or in a feeding chair.[2]

- Open the child's mouth with clean hands and massage the inner cheeks, upper and lower gums, and apply pressure at the tip of the tongue.
- Massage outer cheeks
- Apply pressure at the corners of lips
- Encourage lip closure
- Give a lollipop to suck
- Chewy rubber tubes can be used.[5]

Techniques for Opening the Fist[5]

- Stroke the ulnar side of the hands and fingers.
- Apply pressure at the web between the thumb and index finger.
- Rub the palmar surface with a rough cloth.
- Make the child sit on the ground putting the hands flat on the ground. Tilt the child on one side, so that he presses hard with the palms to break the fall.
- Make the child lean on open hands in sitting and prone position.
- Give play dough in the child's hands.
- Use static cock-up splint.

The journey of bringing up of a child with developmental delay is an uphill task for the parents. We, as a team, need to support them to keep up their motivational level throughout. Our team has got satisfying results with the above-mentioned therapeutic program. However, this is a long drawn out process, and both parents and the therapist need to be patient.

REFERENCES

1. Bobath K, Bobath B. Motor development in the different types of CP, 3rd edition. London: The Whitefriars Press Ltd;1985. pp. 10-2.
2. Spakeman W. Occupational therapy. In: Hopkins HL, Smith HD (Eds). Occupational therapy with children: cerebral palsy. Philadelphia: JB Lippincott Company;1983. pp. 643-81.
3. Bobath B. Tonic neck reflexes and tonic labyrinthine reflexes: abnormal reflex activity caused by brain lesions, 3rd edition. Oxford: Chartered Society of Physiotherapy;1985. pp. 20-37.
4. Manual on Early Intervention in Infants and Toddlers with Developmental Delay. Series 2. Secunderabad: National Institute for the Mentally Handicapped. Shree Ram Processor. 2011. pp. 32-95.
5. Nair MKC. Motor stimulation in infancy. In: The high-risk newborn. Nair MKC (Ed). New Delhi: Jaypee Brothers Medical Publishers; 2008. pp. 282-5.
6. Stamer M. Posture and movement of the child with cerebral palsy. Austin: Therapy Skill Builders under ISBN; 2000. pp. 79-115.
7. Stoppard M. Baby's First Skills. In: Mavle E (Ed). London, New York: Dorling Kinderslay; 2009.pp. 67.

Orthopedic Management in Cerebral Palsy

CHAPTER 8C

Sameer Desai, Rakesh Meena, Ashima Choudhari

INTRODUCTION

Cerebral palsy (CP) results from a static brain lesion during pregnancy or early life. It remains the most common cause of physical disability in children. Spasticity, muscle weakness, and immobility lead to disorders involving muscle, tendons, bones, and joints. Though physiotherapy and occupational therapy form the mainstay of treatment, orthopedic surgical intervention is required for spasticity and contracture management and correcting the lever arms.

DIAGNOSIS AND CLASSIFICATION

The diagnostic matrix to be followed in case of CP includes a detailed history, gait analysis, physical examination of upper and lower limbs, examination of spine, examination under anesthesia, and additional tests for appropriate clinical evaluation.

Gait analysis plays an important part in clinical decision-making when managing children with CP.[1,2] Ambulant children with CP walk with an atypical gait. Optimizing or improving the efficacy of gait is a key orthopedic treatment goal. The various ways in which a clinician can assess gait are as follows:

Visual Observational Gait Analysis

This is performed by assessing body segment motion at the pelvis, hip, knee, and ankle in coronal and sagittal planes and at different points of the gait cycle.

Videographic Gait Analysis

This is performed by observing gait in a slow-motion video and analyzing the joint movements in both planes.

Instrumented Three-dimensional Gait Analysis

The three-dimensional gait analysis (3D GA) has proven to be a particularly powerful and accurate instrument to explicitly quantify joint movements (kinematics) and kinetics of the gait in children with CP. However, 3D GA requires a setup with a lot of expensive infrastructure. Sufficient findings can also be obtained by visual observation and slow-motion videographic gait analysis.

PHYSICAL EXAMINATION OF A CHILD WITH CEREBRAL PALSY

"Observe a child with CP before you touch," this is an important dictum. If the child is apprehensive or tearful, let him stay on the mother's lap while you discuss the birth history with the parents. As the child adapts to the environment, slowly place him on the examination table or on the floor, close to the mother and watch him move around.

The physical examination of the child with CP should include:
- Posture in prone lying, supine lying, sitting, standing, and walking
- Muscle tone of the extremities, trunk and neck, deep tendon reflexes
- Muscle strength
- Range of motion (ROM) at the hip, knee, ankle joints, and foot

TONE

Tone can be defined as resistance to passive stretch, when the muscle is in a relaxed state. In children with CP, tone assessment can be difficult as it is influenced by the child's apprehension and excitement. Depending on the site of brain lesion, the child will present with either spasticity or dystonia. To assess the tone, we need to identify the joint angles during slow, medium, and fast velocities. We also measure the angle where the catch is first felt and also at the end of the joint ROM. The spasticity assessment is commonly done using the modified Tardieu scale and the modified Ashworth scale.

Modified Tardieu Scale

This scale takes into account the resistance to passive movement at both slow and fast speeds. The various parameters that are considered are as follows:
- *R1*: For measuring this, move the muscle group from its shortest to longest position using a rapid velocity stretch. One measures the angle at which muscle resistance or "catch" is felt in response to this rapid stretch.
- *R2*: This measures the maximum passive range of movement of the target muscle group. It is assessed by moving the joint through full ROM using a slow passive movement.

The purpose of the modified Tardieu scale is to measure the spasticity present in a child's muscle and its response to movement. The results can be used to decide which therapeutic interventions should be considered. The difference between angles R1 and R2 gives us an estimate of the presence of spasticity and/or muscle contracture. If there is a large difference between R1 and R2 in outer and middle ROM, it indicates a larger dynamic component. Botulinum toxin A (BTX-A) will be beneficial in a child in this setting. A small difference between R1 and R2 in middle and inner ROM, indicates a fixed contracture and the child will not benefit with a botulinum toxin injection. In such a scenario, the child may require serial casting or surgical lengthening of muscles.

MODIFIED ASHWORTH SCALE

The modified Ashworth scale (MAS) measures resistance during passive soft-tissue stretching and is graded from 0 (no increase in tone) to 4 (affected part rigid in flexion and extension).

Analysis of Range of Motion and Joint Contracture

Assessment of muscle length and joint contractures plays a very important part in the examination of a child with CP. If the examiner feels that the child is not cooperating, then the tests should be repeated at a later date. If required, the measurements should be repeated twice. In some children, examination under anesthesia may be required. The surgeon may have to alter the treatment plan after examining the child under anesthesia. All these findings need to be correlated with history, gait analysis data, and tone assessment.

Hip Joint

Progressive hip dislocation is seen in children with CP. Early detection and appropriate treatment prevents further hip displacement and hip dislocation. Hip dislocation is an important cause of pain, reduced function, and poor quality of life.

Thomas' Hip Flexion Test

This test is commonly used for measuring hip flexion contracture. The child is asked to lie supine on a hard surface. One thigh is flexed with the flexed knee till the exaggerated lumbar lordosis disappears. The angle formed between the horizontal axis of the affected thigh and horizontal line parallel to the floor measures the hip flexion contracture.

Measurement of the Amount of Adductor Contracture

With the patient in supine position, passive abduction of the hip is performed, first with the knee in extension and then with the knee in 90° flexion (Phelps test). When the primary pathology is in the adductor muscles of the hip, then the hip abduction angle in knee flexion and knee extension will be the same. If abduction improves on knee flexion, then the pathology lies in the medial hamstring muscles and gracilis **(Figs. 1A and B)**. A child with decreased hip abduction is likely to have problems during perineal care. Sitting cross-legged becomes very difficult. A child with decreased hip abduction is prone to hip subluxation and dislocation. These children may also exhibit a scissoring gait.

Knee Joint

It is one of the most common joints to be involved. The child may present with fixed flexion deformity or dynamic spasticity of hamstrings. The child may walk in a jump knee gait or crouch gait.

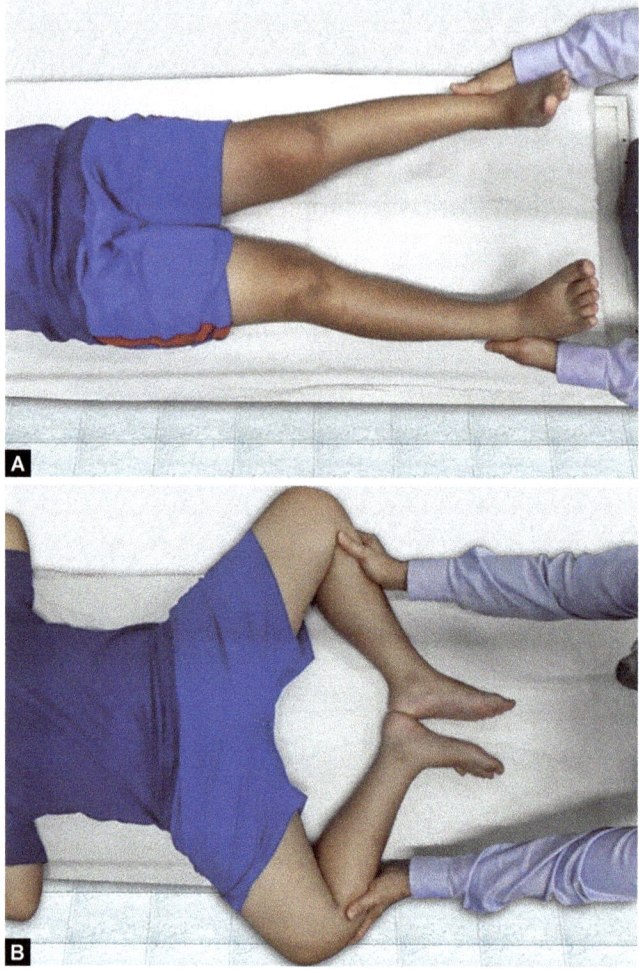

Figs. 1A and B: (A) Hip abduction with knee in extension; (B) Hip abduction with knee in flexion.

Assessment of Rectus Femoris Spasticity

This is measured using the Duncan-Ely/Prone Rectus test.

Assessment of Ankle Equines

Assessment of equines (gastrosoleus spasticity/contracture) is done by passive dorsiflexion of ankle with knee in extension and then with knee joint in 90° flexion (Silfverskiöld test) **(Figs. 2A and B)**. The gastrocnemius muscle crosses the knee joint and flexion is observed as knee relaxes the muscle. If dorsiflexion at ankle increases after flexion at knee joint, then only the gastrocnemius muscle is said to be affected. If dorsiflexion does not increase after knee flexion, then both gastrocnemius and soleus are affected.

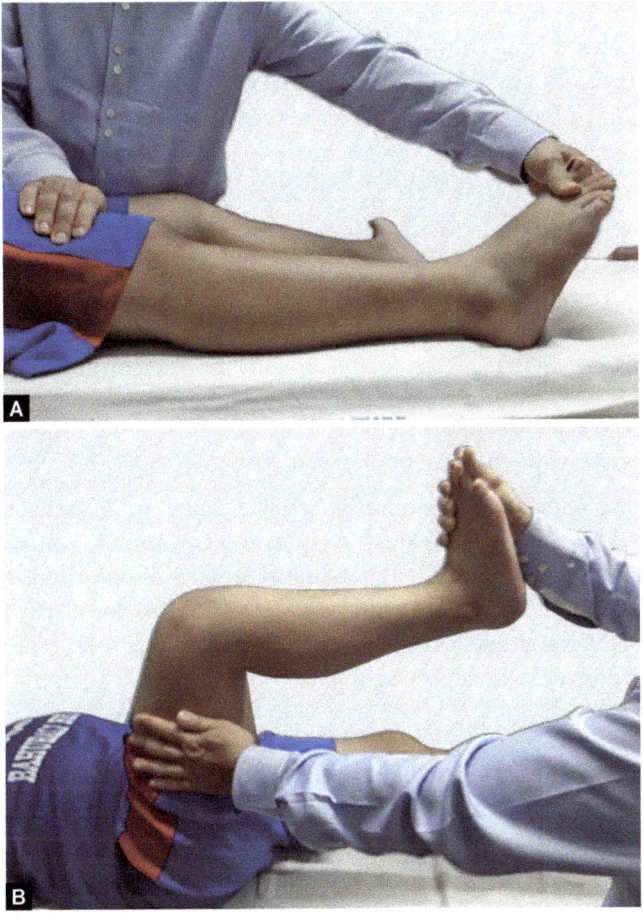

Figs. 2A and B: (A) Ankle dorsiflexion with knee extension (Silfverskiöld test); (B) Ankle dorsiflexion in knee in flexion.

MUSCLE STRENGTH ANALYSIS AND SELECTIVE MOTOR CONTROL

Children with CP typically have decreased muscle strength and lack of selective muscle control. A child with good muscle strength will have good motor function and vice versa. Muscle strength analysis is also required to assess the appropriateness for surgical interventions. In children with CP, the reduced ability to control and isolate movements, provides great hindrance in muscle strength assessment. Tendon transfer will work in children who have good power and selective motor control.

CONCEPT OF LEVER ARM DYSFUNCTION AND TORSIONAL PROFILE

Gage et al.[2] coined the term "Lever arm dysfunction." It is used to describe the particular orthopedic deformities that arise in an ambulatory child with CP. While skeletal structures act as lever arms during walking and muscle activity, the ground reaction against gravity exerts forces on the skeleton. This generates torque (moments) around joints. The common deformities causing lever arm dysfunction in CP are increased femoral anteversion, external tibial torsion, and deformities of the foot.

CLASSIFICATION OF CEREBRAL PALSY

Here we shall see the classifications used by orthopedic surgeons in the management of CP.

The topographic classification of CP is monoplegia, hemiplegia, diplegia, quadriplegia, and triplegia. This classification is helpful to categorize the child in major groups so that we can further classify them according to their gait.

Gait Pattern Classification

Rodda and Graham's Classification System of Spastic Diplegia

The sagittal plane joint movements are considered in this classification.
- *Group I*: True equines. Ankle is in equines. Knee and hip are normal.
- *Group II*: Jump knee. Ankle is in equines. Knee is flexed. Hip is normal.
- *Group III*: Apparent equines. Ankle is normal. Knee is flexed. Hip is normal.
- *Group IV*: Crouch gait. Ankle is in excessive dorsiflexion, knee is flexed, hip is in flexion, and there is pelvic tilt.

Winters and Gage Classification of Hemiplegia[3]

The sagittal plane joint movements are considered in this classification:
- *Group I*: Foot drop during swing phase (apparent equines)
- *Group II*: Persistent ankle dorsiflexion (true equines)
- *Group III*: Child has plantar flexion through gait cycle plus limited knee flexion-extension.
- *Group IV*: In addition to group III, child has reduced hip flexion-extension.

Gross Motor Function Classification System[4]

Using the Gross Motor Function Classification System (GMFCS), the gross motor function of children with CP can be categorized into five different levels. *Level I* being the mildest and *Level V* the most severely affected. This system looks at movements such as sitting, walking, and use of mobility devices. This is an easy method to classify CP which can be used in the outpatient department. It is helpful because it provides clinicians and caregivers with:
- A clear description of a child's current motor function
- An idea of what equipment or mobility aids a child may need in the future, e.g., crutches, walking frames, or wheelchairs

Level I: The child can walk well and climb stairs without using hands for support. The child can run and jump but has decreased speed, balance, and coordination.

Level II: The child can climb stairs holding on to a railing. Walking on uneven surfaces, inclines or in a crowd is difficult for the child. The child can barely run or jump.

Level III: The child can manage to move around indoors and outdoors on level surfaces using assistive mobility devices. The child can propel a manual wheelchair and is able to climb stairs using a railing. However, the child needs assistance for long distances over uneven surfaces.

Level IV: The walking ability is severely limited. The child uses assistive devices such as wheelchairs most of the time. The child may propel own power wheelchair, standing transfers, with or without assistance.

Level V: The child has physical impairments in the form of very poor head, neck, and trunk control, infact in all areas of motor function. Even with adaptive equipment, the child cannot sit or stand independently.

MUSCULOSKELETAL PATHOLOGY MANAGEMENT

The primary aim in the management of children with CP is to prevent the development of deformities by following a good physiotherapy protocol and by prescribing braces. Spasticity is one of the positive features of the "upper motor neuron" syndrome and is associated with co-contraction, clonus, and hyperreflexia. The negative features of the upper-motor neuron syndrome (weakness, loss of selective motor control, and sensory impairment) are also important and may have a greater impact on function and prognosis than the positive features. Once spasticity and contractures have set in, we may need to reestablish the balance of muscle forces. This can be achieved by injecting BTX-A in target muscles or by performing soft tissue releases, tendon transfers, and bony reconstructions. Treatment goals should be individualized and consistent with expected benefits. The goals of management vary according to the level of the brain lesion, topographical classification, GMFCS, functional mobility score of the child, and complicating factors such as epilepsy. For a patient with GMFCS IV and V, the treatment goals are improving nursing care, hygiene, and improving sitting balance by having well-located and painless hips and a straight spine. For a child with GMFCS I, II, and III, the goals will be to improve gait and make it more energy efficient. Thus, orthopedic interventions in CP can be broadly categorized into:
- Correct deformity—static or dynamic
- Balance muscle power
- Stabilize uncontrollable joints

BOTULINUM TOXIN A

Botulinum toxin A is one of the seven different serotypes of botulinum toxin (A-G) produced by the anaerobic bacterium *Clostridium* botulinum.[5,6] BTX-A has been commercially available with different names (Botox, Dysport) for clinical use for a long time. It should be noted that it also has to be considered as one of the strongest poisons of the world and is potentially lethal if not used in a safe way. Spasticity is an important feature of CP because it contributes to reduced muscle growth and impairment of function. This in turn leads to progressive musculoskeletal deformity and fixed contractures. BTX-A is one of the important modalities in the treatment of children with spasticity.

Mechanism of Action

After BTX-A has been injected directly into the muscle, it is selectively taken up by endocytosis at the cholinergic nerve terminal, where it blocks the release of acetylcholine. A temporary reduced muscular activity (chemical denervation) occurs in the injected muscle. This process is reversible and recovery is possible due to terminal sprouting and definitive repair. The elimination of the sprouts results in the return of synaptic function to the original neuromuscular junction. This requires about 91 days. The period of clinically useful relaxation is usually seen between 3 and 24 weeks.

Dosage

Although BTX-A has a high potential therapeutic value as a tone reducer, safe recommended total dosages recently reported in the literature for children are shown in **Table 1**.

Indication and Usage

- Focal spasticity due to CP in children
- Other uses are management of blepharospasm, cervical dystonia, hemifacial spasm, focal dystonia, hyperkinetic facial lines, drooling of saliva, etc.

Method of Administration

After adequate dilution in normal saline, BTX-A is directly injected in target muscle belly at various sites. Some of the common muscles are gastrocnemius, hamstrings, psoas, pronator, and wrist flexors. The muscle can be identified by direct palpation, using ultrasound guidance or by electromyography of the muscle. These special methods are especially useful while targeting muscles of upper limb.

Post-BTX-A Protocol

In lower limb, the child may require single or multiple plasters to stretch the contracted muscles. Plaster is not preferred for upper limb. Physiotherapy is started once the child becomes comfortable and cooperative.

TABLE 1: Dosage of botulinum toxin A.

	Botox	Dysport
Range (U/kg)	1–20	1–20
Maximum total dose (U)	400–600	500–1,000
Range maximum dose/site (U)	10–50	50–250

Side Effects

Increasing the dose of BTX-A brings an increased potential for adverse side effects. Localized side effects of BTX-A are consequences of muscle relaxation, such as weakness or initial loss of function which can occur as patients learn to readjust their postural control in response to altered muscle tone. Systemic side effects due to spread of toxin beyond the site of injection are asthenia, generalized muscle weakness, diplopia, ptosis, blurred vision, facial weakness, swallowing and speech disorders, constipation, aspiration pneumonia, dysphagia, and urinary incontinence.

Advantages

Botulinum toxin A can be seen as a valuable treatment option within the variety of tone-reduction treatments, because it can reduce muscle tone, is safe at a young age, reversible, selective, allows combined treatment, and is dose-dependent. BTX-A gives the physiotherapist a window period to strengthen the antagonist muscles and to stretch the spastic muscles. It also improves brace compliance and decreases pain.

Disadvantages

High financial cost and reversible action lead to requirement of repeated injections.

ORTHOPEDIC SURGICAL INTERVENTION

Foot Problems

Foot disorders are the most common problems in children with CP. The natural history of the deformities of the feet is variable and unpredictable. In the initial period, the children should be treated with orthotics and manual therapy. Some common problems are:

- *Equines*: It is due to tendo-Achilles contracture **(Fig. 3)**. The child will walk on the toes and is seen in true equines and jump knee gait. BTX-A is usually injected in this muscle.[7] If there is a severe contracture, then surgical lengthening is performed after 8 years of age. Low tendo-Achilles lengthening and isolated tendo-Achilles lengthening should not be performed as it leads to excessive weakness and crouch gait.
- *Equinovarus*: The foot points downward and inward. It may also develop because of spastic tibialis anterior and posterior in addition to spastic tendo-Achilles, which may require botulinum toxin injection, lengthening, or tendon transfer.
- *Equinovalgus*: The foot points downward and outward. It happens due to tight tendo-Achilles and midfoot break. Bilateral planovalgus deformity often improves till the age of 5 or 6 years. It is stable in middle childhood, but worsens later on. It becomes painful during adolescence. The primary treatment should always be orthotic control. In the initial period, the child is given orthotics to control the foot position during gait. Later, it often

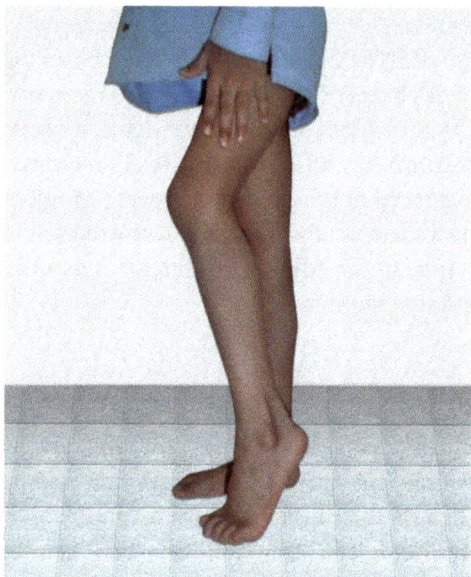

Fig. 3: Child with spasticity of left tendo-Achilles.

requires lateral calcaneal lengthening (Mosca procedure) or fusion of foot bones (extra-articular arthrodesis).

- *Hallux valgus*: The big toe points toward and sometimes under the second toe. It is usually associated with valgus deformity of foot. Hallux valgus can be corrected by a proximal resection to the bunion and a phalangeal osteotomy. Ambulatory patients may be treated with great toe metatarsophalangeal joint arthrodesis using a small plate and screw.

KNEE FLEXION DEFORMITY (FIG. 4)

Flexed-knee gait, which is defined by abnormally high knee flexion, is the most common pattern of gait deformity in the CP population.[8] The factors are many and interlinked. These include torsional malalignments, abnormal motor control, muscle weakness and imbalance, muscle contractures, spasticity, and foot deformities. The child may have crouch gait because of additional tendo-Achilles weakness. These children are usually treated with single event multilevel surgery which includes hamstring lengthening and supracondylar extension osteotomy of femur along with patellar tendon shortening. In addition, we may have to address other joints too.

HIP SUBLUXATION AND DISLOCATION (FIG. 5)

Hip displacement is the second most common musculoskeletal problem in children with CP.[9] Hip displacement is not related to the movement disorder but is related directly to gross motor function as determined by the GMFCS. The incidence is more in GMFCS IV and V.

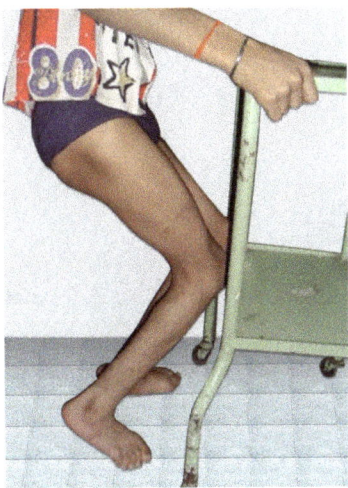

Fig. 4: Child with crouch gait.

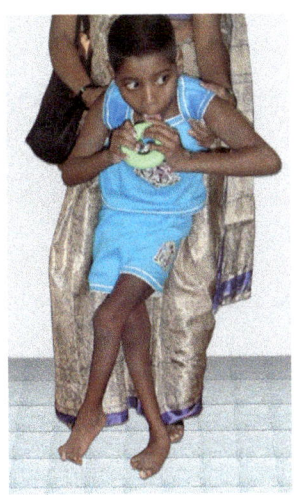

Fig. 5: Child with scissoring and right hip dislocation.

Hip Surveillance[10,11]

Early identification and treatment prevents progressive hip displacement and its sequelae such as pain and difficulty in squatting. Children with CP have enlocated hips at birth. However, in some children, they progress rapidly to hip subluxation and dislocation. This can be monitored using anterior-posterior (AP) pelvis X-ray. On serial radiographs, we measure the migration percentage (MP). A MP >30% is referred to as being subluxated. When MP is >50%, then hip is labeled as dislocated. Initial clinical assessment and AP pelvic radiograph is always advised at 12-24 months of age. The frequency of radiographs is determined by GMFCS level, radiological measures, and clinical assessment. Ideally, radiographs are performed every 6 months to 1 year till 4 years. If migration percentage is stable, then further reviews are done at 4 years, 7 years, and again at skeletal maturity. If migration percentage is increasing, then repeated radiographs are advised every 6-12 months till skeletal maturity.

Management

Interventions to prevent or manage hip displacement in children with CP vary depending on the MP and GMFCS of the child. In a younger child, injections of botulinum neurotoxin, bracing, phenolization of the obturator nerve, and adductor releases are performed. In an older child, or a child with hip dislocation, femoral osteotomies, pelvic osteotomies, and salvage procedures are required.

SCOLIOSIS

Scoliosis is common in children with CP. It is estimated that scoliosis occurs in between 21 and 64% of patients with CP. This is seen mainly in quadriplegics and nonambulatory children. A child with scoliosis can have associated

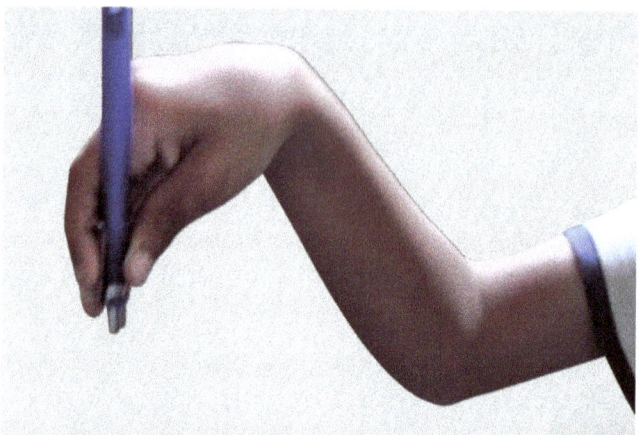

Fig. 6: Child with deformity of hand.

kyphosis or lordosis. The progression of the curve depends on the severity of CP and can continue even beyond skeletal maturity. Curves of smaller magnitude (Cobb's angle <20) need follow-up with serial radiographs. In early cases (Cobb's angle 20–50°), a brace can be given to improve sitting balance or to slow the rate of curve progression. However, for larger curves (Cobb's angle > 50°), surgery may be required. The aim of surgery is to improve sitting balance and prevent hip subluxation. The commonly used implants are screws and wires along with rod system.

Upper Limb

Finger flexion, wrist flexion, thumb adduction, elbow flexion and shoulder adduction, and internal rotation are the common deformities seen in these children[12] **(Fig. 6)**. Occupational therapy and physiotherapy are important to improve hand function. Management of hemiplegic hand is more difficult as child adapts to using the normal hand, and it is very difficult to break the abnormal pattern. Treatment with BTX-A has a small effect in the upper limb and the action is short-lived. Children with higher levels of function may benefit from various combinations of muscle–tendon lengthening for flexion deformities and tendon transfers and for muscle imbalance, joint stabilization, and correction of "thumb-in-palm" deformity. In severe deformity, wrist fusion may be required. Another common surgery that is performed is transfer of flexor carpi ulnaris to extensor carpi radialis brevis to improve persistent wrist palmer flexion during the grip. This transfer improves the grip strength. The outcomes of surgical management are greater than those obtained from physiotherapy or botulinum toxin.

REFERENCES

1. Stéphane A, Geraldo D, Bonnefoy-Mazure A. Gait analysis in children with cerebral palsy. Effort Open Rev. 2016;1(12):448-60.
2. Gage JR, Schwartz MH, Koop SE, Novacheck TF. The identification and treatment of gait problems in cerebral palsy. London: Mac Keith Press; 2009.

3. Winters TF, Gage JR, Hicks R. Gait patterns in spastic hemiplegia in children and young adults. J Bone Joint Surg Am. 1987;69(3):437-41.
4. Palisano RJ, Rosenbaum PL, Walter S, Russell D, Wood E, Galuppi B. Development and reliability of a system to classify gross motor function in child with cerebral palsy. Dev Med Child Neurol.1997;39(4):214-23.
5. Franzén M, Hägglund G, Alriksson-Schmidt A. Treatment with botulinum toxin A in a total population of children with cerebral palsy: a retrospective cohort registry study. BMC Musculoskelet Disord. 2017;18:520.
6. Bjornson K, Hays R, Graubert C, Price R, Won F, McLaughlin JF, et al. Botulinum toxin for spasticity in children with cerebral palsy: a comprehensive evaluation. Pediatrics. 2007;120(1):49-58.
7. Kelly B, MacKay-LyonsMJ, Berryman S, Hyndman J, WoodE. Assessment protocol for serial casting after botulinum toxin A injections to treat equinus gait. Pediatr Phys Ther. 2008;20(3):233-41.
8. Rodda JM, Graham HK, Nattrass GR, Galea MP, Baker R, Wolfe R. Correction of severe crouch gait in patients with spastic diplegia with use of multilevel orthopaedic surgery. J Bone Joint Surg Am. 2006;88(12):2653-64.
9. Bagg MR, Farber J, Miller F. Long-term follow-up of hip subluxation in cerebral palsy patients. J Pediatr Orthop.1993;13(1):32-6.
10. Wynter M, Gibson N, Kentish M, Love S, Thomason P, Graham HK. The Consensus Statement on Hip Surveillance for Children with Cerebral Palsy: Australian Standards of Care. J Pediatr Rehabil Med. 2011;4(3):183-95.
11. Gordon G, Simkiss DE. A systematic review of the evidence for hip surveillance in children with cerebral palsy. J Bone Joint Surg Br. 2006;88(11):1492-6.
12. Holmström L, Vollmer B, Tedroff K, Islam M, Persson JK, Kits A, et al. Hand function in relation to brain lesions and corticomotor projection pattern in children with unilateral cerebral palsy. Dev Med Child Neurol. 2010;52(2):145-52.

CHAPTER 9

Learning Disabilities in Low Birth Weight Children

Sudha Chaudhari

INTRODUCTION

Many low birth weight children appear quite normal in early childhood. However, they show many cognitive problems when they enter school, specifically learning disabilities (LDs). These consist of difficulties in reading, writing, and mathematics. They may not be obvious early on in Kindergarten, but are apparent in third or fourth standard when academic skills become demanding.

The term learning disability was first described by Kirk in 1962. These consist of difficulties in learning:
- Inaccurate or slow word reading with a lot of effort
- Difficulty in understanding the meaning of what is read
- Difficulty with spelling and written expression
- Difficulty in mastering number sense, numerical facts or calculations and mathematical reasoning, and inability to apply any concepts

Thus, the affected academic skills are substantially lower than those expected for their chronologic age and significantly affect their academic, occupational performance, and activities of daily living.[1] It should be confirmed that these difficulties are not accounted by intellectual disabilities, uncorrected visual or auditory acuity, psychosocial adversity, language problems, or inadequate educational instructions.

INCIDENCE

The incidence of LD is reported more in boys than girls.[2] Tanabe reported that very low birth weight (VBLW) and intrauterine growth restriction posed a high risk of LD in children born in Japan.[3] Litt reported a high rate of specifically mathematics LD in extremely low birth weight (ELBW) children at adolescence, compared to their normal peers.[4]

The diagnosis of LD should be made based on a synthesis of the child's history (developmental, medical, family, and education), school reports, and psychosocial assessment.

READING DISORDER (DYSLEXIA)

The children have impairment in: (1) word reading accuracy, (2) the rate of reading or fluency, and (3) reading comprehension. Children with reading disorder (RD) have difficulties with phonologic processing: the process of identifying and manipulating individual sounds (phonemes) with larger sound units (morphemes and words). Problems with phonological processing are noticed in the preschool age, but never definitely identified till early school age. Rickards et al.[5] found that 24% of their VLBW cohort had not achieved reading accuracy at 14 years, and 48% had not reached the criterion for reading comprehension. Thus, dyslexic children have a pattern of learning difficulties that is characterized by problems with accurate or fluent word recognition, poor decoding, and poor spelling abilities. They may have difficulties in reading with additional difficulties in comprehension or mathematics reasoning.

DISORDER OF WRITTEN EXPRESSION (DYSGRAPHIA)

The key feature of a disorder of written expression is a markedly reduced ability to organize and present information in writing compared with a stronger ability to organize and present information in the oral–verbal modality. They lack spelling accuracy **(Fig. 1)**. They also lack clarity or organization of written expression. Dysgraphia will not become apparent till the child reaches a higher grade, since the 5- or 6-year-old children have limited writing demands, and do not need significant development of ideas or use of grammar. It is only in the third or fourth standard that parents and teachers realize that the child has a writing problem.

A study from Finland[6] showed that the premies achieved lower scores than full-term controls in writing. In our study,[7] 25% of VLBW children had significantly poorer writing skills compared with 6.7% in normal controls.

MATHEMATICS DISORDER (DYSCALCULIA)

These children lack number sense, memorization of arithmetic facts and accurate mathematics reasoning, and accurate calculations. They have difficulties in mental calculation and over-rely on memory and tangible aids **(Fig. 2)**.

Table 1 shows the comparison between the mathematical skills and of the low birth weight (LBW) group and the control group in the 'Pune Low Birth Weight Study'.

The LBW group had a mean score of 82.7 ± 16.9, which was significantly less than that of the control group.[7] When the scores were compared according to birth weight categories, the VLBW children had a significantly lower score. When comparison was made by weight for gestation age, the preterm small for gestation age (SGA) children had a significantly lower score.

These impairments may be mild, in learning social skills, and in one or two domains. The child may be able to compensate/function well with adequate support in the school years. In the moderate LD group, there may be marked difficulties in learning skills in one or more academic domains. They are unlikely to function well without intensive and specialized teaching during school years. In the severe variety, the child has major difficulties in learning skills and needs remedial teaching throughout the school years.

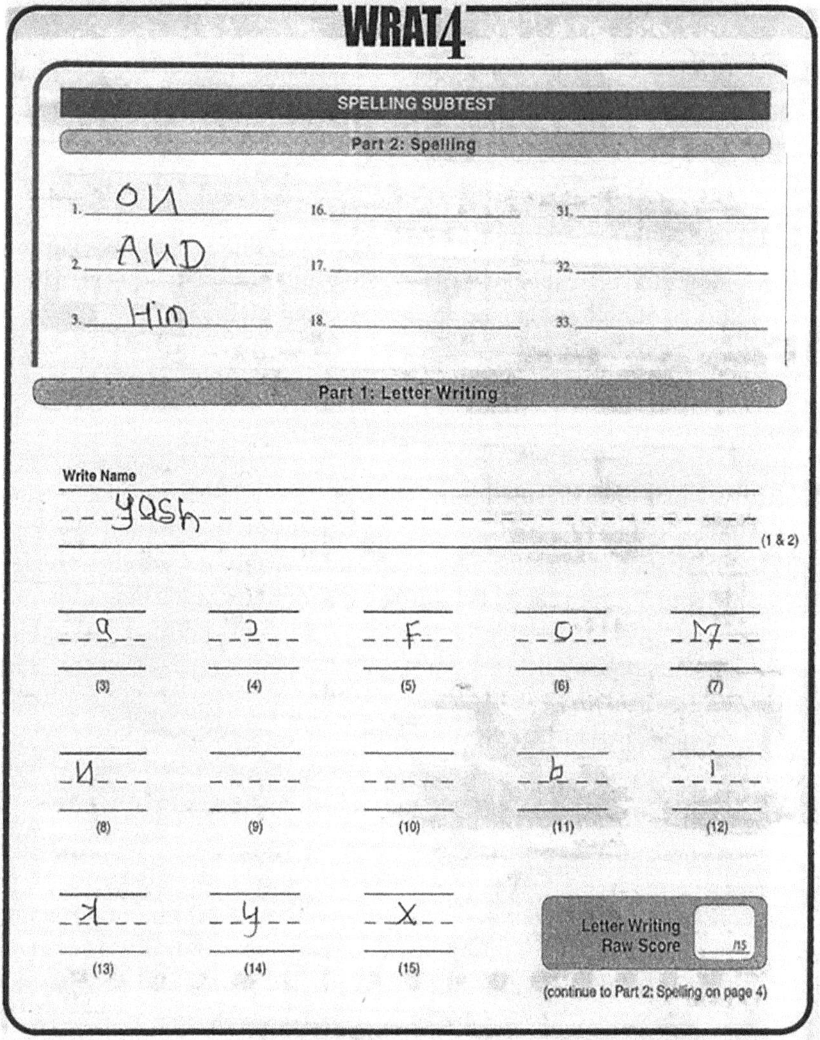
WRAT4

SPELLING SUBTEST

Part 2: Spelling

1. ON 16. 31.

2. AND 17. 32.

3. Him 18. 33.

Part 1: Letter Writing

Write Name

yash (1 & 2)

(3) (4) (5) (6) (7)

(8) (9) (10) (11) (12)

(13) (14) (15)

Letter Writing Raw Score /15

(continue to Part 2: Spelling on page 4)

Fig. 1: Dysgraphia.

Isaacs et al.[8] investigated the neural bases of LD in preterm infants by using a neuroimaging modality. They did voxel-based morphometry of adolescent children born with gestation <31 weeks, to investigate the relationship between brain structure and a specific LD. There is no overactivation of left occipito-temporal region even after repeated trials of word exposure in dyslexic children. As they grow older, they show overactivation of left inferior frontal gyrus **(Figs. 3 and 4)**. Isaacs found that there is a specific area in the parietal lobe where the children without dyscalculia have more gray matter than those with dyscalculia.

Breslau[9] showed that LBW children at the age of 17 years were approximately 50% more likely to have reading and mathematics problems compared to normal birth weight children. Saigal et al.[10] reported similar results in a study

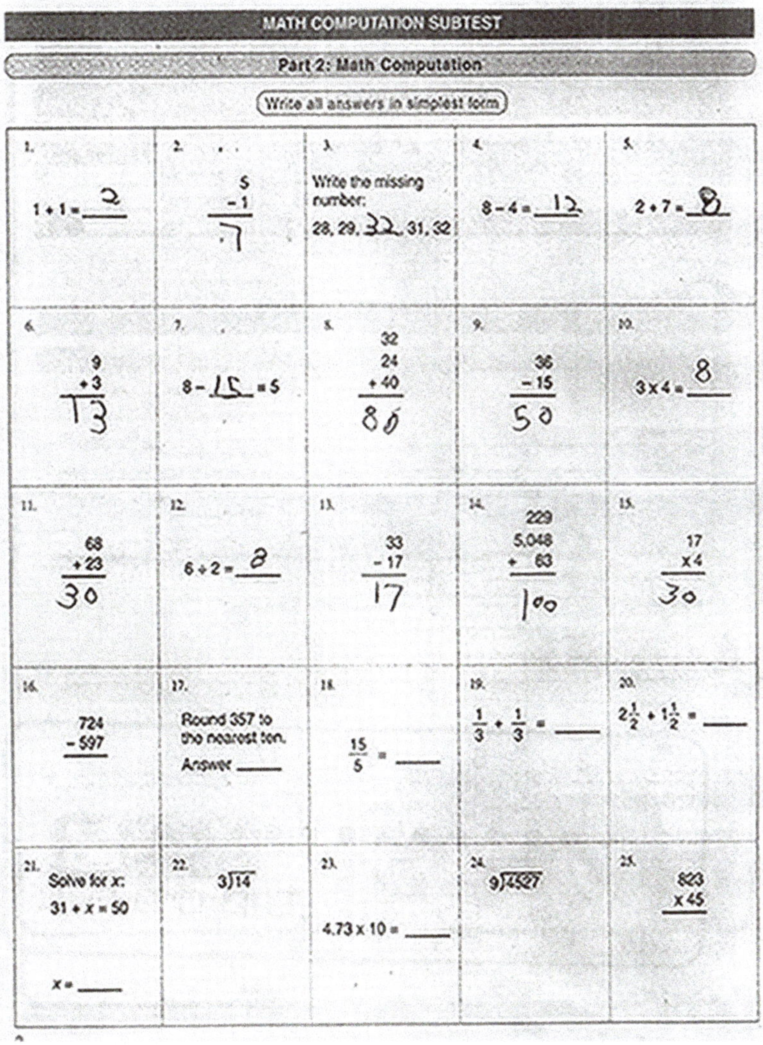

Fig. 2: Dyscalculia.

TABLE 1: Comparison of mathematics score (WRAT) between LBW and controls at 12 years.

Groups	n	Mathematics Score Mean (SD)
All LBW	180	82.7 (16.9)*
Birthweight <1,500 g	78	80.4 (15.1)**
Birthweight 1,500–1,999 g	102	84.4 (17.9)
Preterm SGA	73	81.6 (18.0)*
Full term SGA	33	82.7 (16.2)
Preterm AGA	74	83.7 (16.1)
Controls	90	87.8 (15.8)

*$p<0.01$, **$p<0.001$
(AGA: appropriate for gestational age; LBW: low birth weight; SGA: small for gestational age; WRAT: Wide Range of Achievement Test)

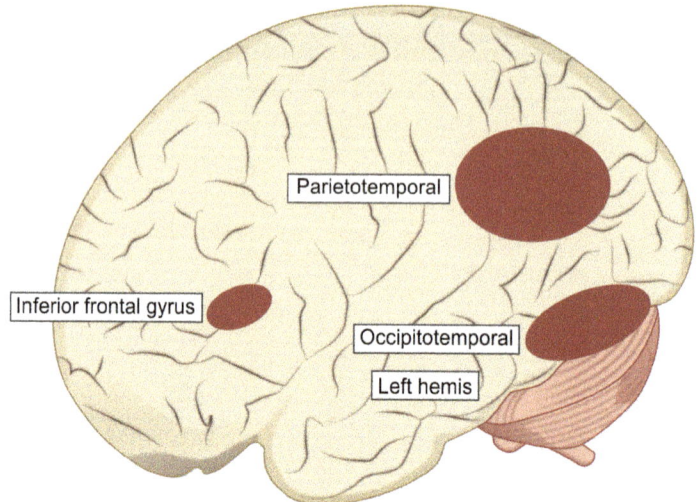

Fig. 3: Normal reading with anterior and posterior activation.

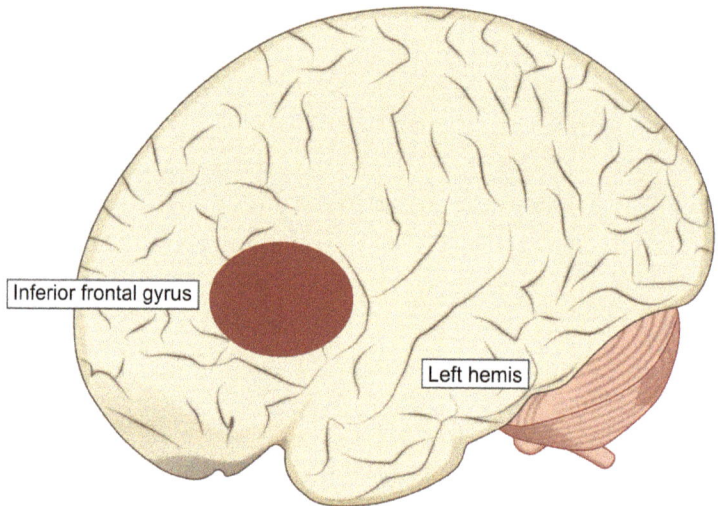

Fig. 4: Overactivation in a reader with dyslexia.

spanning four countries—USA, Canada, Holland, and Bavaria at the ages of 8–11 years.

A dyslexic phenotype with deficits in phonologic awareness has been linked to chromosome 6. History of dyslexia in a family member is a significant risk factor.

PREDICTION

With the fast increase in the survival of VLBW and ELBW infants, parents and neonatologists have increasing concern about the academic potential of these neonatal intensive care unit (NICU) graduates. In order to achieve good academic outcome, these children have to be identified early.

Saigal et al.[11] tried to identify LD[1] in ELBW children using a kindergarten screening battery at 5 years. The children were reassessed at 8 years using the Wide Range of Achievement Test 4 (WRAT-4) and found that the prediction done at 5 years was poor. She also looked at the effect of maternal education on reading, spelling, and mathematics at 8 years. In our study,[12] although maternal education was very important, it was the father's education that was important for both writing and mathematics in a regression model. A second important factor contributing to the variance was the type of school attended by the child, a factor hitherto not reported in any studies.

IMPORTANCE OF EARLY DIAGNOSIS

Preschool identification of specific learning disability (SLD) is difficult. It is important to identify a specific LD as early as possible. The longer the child goes without remediation, the lower the rate of success.

Wide Range of Achievement Test 4 (WRAT-4)

It is an achievement test which measures an individual's ability to read words, comprehend sentences, spell words, and compute solutions to mathematics problems. WRAT-4 is used as a measure of basic academic skills necessary for effective learning, reading, and spelling words and performing basic mathematical calculation. Age group—5 years onward.

Wechsler's Individual Achievement Test III (WIAT-III) 2005

WIAT-III assesses the academic achievement of children above 4 years. It has a total of 16 subtests in the areas of listening, speaking, reading, writing, and mathematical skills.

Woodcock–Johnson IV Test of Achievement 2014

It is a test for individual evaluation of academic achievements, cognitive ability and oral language, and to identify learning problems. Age group—preschool to adulthood.

RED FLAG SIGNS FOR LEARNING DISABILITIES

- Family history of reading delay
- Early delayed talking—first word after 15 months, phrases after 24 months
- Pronunciation difficulties after 5–6 years
- Difficulty attending to sound of words, confusing words that sound alike
- Delayed establishment of laterality
- Difficulty in fine motor skills
- Clumsy child

Low birth weight children should be referred early before significant reading delays occur. They need a multidisciplinary team of specialists: (1) A developmental pediatrician, (2) Psychologist, (3) Speech therapist, and (4) Special educator. The neurodevelopmental pediatrician takes a detailed history and does a physical examination. In a majority of LD children, this examination is normal except for a few soft neurologic signs. The psychologist does a standard IQ test and establishes the child's normal intelligence. This will help exclude poor home and school environment or other stressors for the child's poor performance like borderline intelligence, or mild mental retardation as the causes of LD. The most commonly used test is WRAT, which tests all three skills—reading, writing, and mathematics.[12]

TREATMENT

Intervention is offered to young children to improve their reading skills. The services of a special educator will definitely be needed, and she will prepare an Individualized Education Plan (IEP) for the specific LD. Although it is rare to completely outgrow the academic weakness, their performance in the special area can be improved markedly with special interventions.

Being an invisible handicap, there are no national guidelines in India for certification of SLD. The recommendations vary from state to state. However, some facilities such as extra time, vocational subjects instead of third language or algebra, and geometry are given in the board examinations.

REFERENCES

1. American Psychiatric Association. Diagnostic and Statistical Manual of Mental Disorders, 5th edition. (DSM 5). New York: CBS Publishers and Distributors; 2011. pp. 66-74.
2. Olitsky SE, Nelson LB. Reading disorders in children. Pediatr Clin North Am. 2003;50(1):213-24.
3. Tanabe K, Tamakoshi K, Kirkmuchi, Murotsuki J. Learning disability in 10–16 year old adolescents with very low birth weight in Japan. 2014;232(1):27-33.
4. Litt J, Taylor HG, Klein N, Hack M. Learning disabilities in children with very low birthweight: prevalence, neuropsychological correlates, and educational interventions. J Learn Disabil. 2005;38(2):130-41.
5. Rickards AL, Kelly EA, Doyle LW, Callanan C. Cognitive, behavioural and academic progress in very low birth-weight (VLBW) children to 14 years of age. J Paediar Child Health. 1998;34:Abstract.
6. LuomaL, Herrgard BN, Martikainen AL. Neuropsychological analysis of the visuomotor problems in children born preterm at <32 weeks of gestation: a 5-year prospective follow-up. Developmental Medicine and Child Neurology. 1998;40(1):21-30.
7. Chaudhari S, Otiv M, Chitale A, Pandit A, Hoge M. Pune low birth weight study: cognitive abilities and educational performance at twelve years. Indian Pediatr. 2004;41(2):121-8.
8. Isaacs EB, Edmonds CJ, Lucas A, Gadian DG. Calculation difficulties in children of very low birthweight: a neural correlate. Brain. 2001;124(Pt 9):1701-7.
9. Breslau N, Paneth NS, Lucia VC. The lingering academic deficits of low birth weight children. Pediatrics. 2004;114(4):1035-40.
10. Saigal S, den Ouden L, Wolke D, Hoult L, Paneth N, Streiner DL, et al. School-age outcomes in children who were extremely low birth weight from four international population-based cohorts. Pediatrics. 2003;112(4):943-50.
11. Saigal S, Szatmari P, Rasenbaum P. Can learning disabilities in children who were extremely low birth weight be identified at school entry? Dev and Behav Ped. 1992;13(5):356-61.
12. Chaudhari S, Otiv M, Chitale A, Hoge M, Pandit A, Mote A. Biology versus environment in low birth weight children. Indian Pediatr. 2005;42(8):763-70.

Parenting a Child with Disability

Sudha Chaudhari

INTRODUCTION

It is extremely stressful for the parents to care for a child who is high-risk and later may develop a disability. Four types of specific reactions are seen when parents have a high-risk or premature infant.[1]

1. *The immediate reaction:* The first reaction that these parents will have is fear that the child may die. The parents are most anxious because they cannot be with their precious baby after transfer to the neonatal intensive care unit (NICU). They become particularly anxious when the baby is being ventilated. Those mothers who have conceived through in vitro fertilization (IVF) are heartbroken because they have waited so long to have a healthy baby.

    These feelings recede after a few weeks, but then the complaint game begins. They complain about the busy nursing staff who has been late in giving the tube feed, about the nursing staff being rude. They constantly ask the staff about the condition of the baby every few hours and complain that the resident doctors are noncommunicative. After a stay of few weeks in the NICU, financial problems crop up, which increases their stress. In order to decrease the anxiety of the parents, at the KEM Hospital, Pune, we have a fixed time for a daily counseling session by the consultant in charge. The social worker also attends this session to sort out monetary and other problems. We encourage parents, grandparents, and any other close relatives to attend the session, so they can ask their queries and their fears can be allayed.

2. Once the discharge is imminent, they become very anxious about how they will be able to handle such a tiny baby. They will repeatedly ask questions about apnea, temperature control, whether they need room heaters in winter, whether they can use air-conditioning in summer. A short stay of 3 or 4 days in the "step down nursery" under the supervision of a nurse boosts their self-confidence. Those parents who have come from other far off cities are worried about the transport and journey. After going home, the overanxious mother may spend sleepless nights, which may affect her breast milk output.

3. Diagnosing a disability is a slow process in the first year and parents have to be told in a gentle manner about the possibility of delayed development. Many parents have great difficulty in dealing with uncertainty.[2] The parents may question the physician's diagnosis and will seek a second opinion.

We should support this decision of the parents and help them to get another opinion and not be upset by their lack of faith in you, and lose interest in the child.

In preterm infants, because of the transient nature of the many tone abnormalities, one tends to defer the diagnosis. Some parents cannot accept this uncertainty and feel that the physician is not telling them the truth. The parents should be frequently updated on the current neurologic status of the baby.

4. *Emotional reaction to diagnosis of disability*: Grief is first felt when they see a scrawny low birth weight child. Parents are also saddened by the pain and struggle the child has to face, the many painful visits for assessments and therapy.[3] The intensity of the sorrow may decrease over a period of time, but becomes more poignant during birthdays, festivals, when they are surrounded by other normal children.

The mother frequently faces guilt and feels that it is her fault that she delivered a premature baby. This is compounded by the fact that the husband or mother-in-law start blaming her.

Parenting a "special child" is a full time and demanding job for the mother. So, if the father can take over for a few hours after coming back from the office, the mother can relax and have some "me time."

In many instances, the husband's family does not even come and visit this baby in the hospital, especially if it is a girl child and many marriages have broken up because of this issue. There may be anger and rejection towards the infant who is irritable and makes overwhelming demands. Some parents resent the change in their lifestyle because of the demands of the disabled child.

The "Vulnerable Child Syndrome" was first reported by Green and Solnit in 1964.[4] This syndrome describes the behavioral and developmental patterns that emerge from aberrations of parenting styles. The predisposing factors in the parents are: (1) previous miscarriage, sudden infant death, or intrauterine deaths, (2) IVF baby, and (3) serious and life-threatening illness in the NICU, when the physician may have discussed impending death. This may result in overprotectiveness where the mother restricts the child's activities and contacts with other children and adults for fear of infection. She does not entrust the care of the child to anybody else. Giving into the child's excessive demands, overindulgence and overprotectiveness, results in a completely stubborn and spoilt child. This style of parenting is detrimental to the social and emotional development of the child. The parents' inability to set limits and encourage independence results in poor peer relations, separation anxieties, and lack of self-confidence. Counseling the parents in such a situation is very important.

When the child with a disability grows up, the most important skill he or she must develop is a strong sense of self-worth and self-esteem. The child should be encouraged to be as independent as possible and overindulgence should be avoided. Siblings should be encouraged to accept and adjust to this child. Parents should be counseled to balance attention to other siblings and not obsess over the "special" child.

REFERENCES

1. Minde K. Parenting the premature infant: Problems and opportunities. In: Taeusch HW, Yogman MW (Eds). Follow-up Management of the High-Risk Infant. Boston, Little Brown, 1987, pp. 315-22.
2. Amiel-Tison C, Grenier A. Neurologic assessment during the first year of life. New York: Oxford University Press. 1986; pp. 6-9.
3. Bernbaum J, Hoffman-Williamson M. Primary care of the preterm infant. Philadelphia: Mosby Year Book. 1991;pp.283-5.
4. Beckwith L. Adverse reaction. In: Taeusch HW, Yogman MW (Eds). Follow-up Management of the High-Risk Infant. Boston, Little Brown, 1987, pp. 323-7.

Pune Low Birth Weight Study: Birth to 22 Years

Sudha Chaudhari

INTRODUCTION

The survival of "high-risk" neonates has improved considerably with better perinatal care. But mere survival is not enough; it is the quality of survival that is important. In 1982, we started a 24-bed neonatal unit at KEM Hospital. It was the largest neonatal unit in the city at that time, admitting inborn and outborn babies. However, there was no data in India about the neurodevelopment of these babies. So, a long-term follow-up of these high-risk infants was planned. We were fortunate because we had started the TDH Rehabilitation and Morris Child Development Centre on the floor below. This center had all the facilities needed for a follow-up and therapy of high-risk newborns. So we started a long-term follow-up of our neonatal intensive care unit (NICU) graduates and this entire 22-year study was done in five phases. It was funded by Indian Council of Medical Research (ICMR), New Delhi, and conducted at KEM Hospital, Pune. Though this is a study from the preventilation era, when very few extremely low birth weight (ELBW) babies were being saved, the methodology is worth emulating. In an era, where the incidence of type II diabetes is sky rocketing in India, the 22-year follow-up, where predictors of "metabolic syndrome" were studied, would be of great interest. This chapter gives a summary of the findings in the 22 years follow-up of low birth weight (LBW) newborns.

PHASE I

An In-depth Longitudinal Study of Development of High-risk Neonates from 0 to 30 Months

Neurodevelopment is a multiphasic and multidimensional phenomenon. The vulnerable, helpless, extremely dependent neonate changes into a mobile, independent child with a mind of its own. This transformation is influenced not only by factors or risks at or soon after birth, but by several external influences such as family and social environment. So a multidisciplinary approach, with close collaboration of the neonatologist, psychologist, occupational therapist, social worker, audiologist, and ophthalmologist was developed and a High Risk Clinic (HRC) was started two times a week. Infants admitted between October 1987 and April 1989 with the following risk factors were enrolled.

- Birth weight <2 kg.
- Gestation <37 weeks
- *Birth asphyxia*: Apgar score <5 at 5 minutes

- Hyperbilirubinemia
- Septicemia/meningitis
- Intraventricular hemorrhage
- Seizures
- *Respiratory distress:* Mild, moderate, and severe on Silverman's score
- Apnea

Babies, discharged from the postnatal ward with birth weight >2,500 g with a normal antenatal, natal, and postnatal course, born during the same period were enrolled as controls.

At the time of discharge, a specially prepared green card was given. The importance of a regular follow-up was explained to the parents. The paternal grandmother was especially called at this time, because mother-in-laws play an important role in decisions regarding child rearing in our society. The social worker, who already had a close rapport with the family because she interacted with them everyday in the NICU, gathered all the information about the family, their income, housing, and education level, etc. Socioeconomic status of the family was determined by the Kuppuswamy Scale.

A simple stimulation program was advised. The parents were asked to hang a mobile on the cradle. They were told to use a "pooja bell" for auditory stimulation and a red ball for visual stimulation. Soft music was recommended, whenever the baby woke up for a feed.

All neurological and psychological assessments were done during the clinic visits. Immunization was also done during the clinic visit. A letter was sent 1 week before the appointment for testing, as a reminder for parents. If an appointment was missed, a home visit was made by the social worker to find out the cause for defaulting. Thus, an all-out effort was made to minimize hospital visits.

When the baby came to the HRC, anthropometric measurements were taken, and a physical examination was done. Intercurrent illnesses were treated. If treatment was taken elsewhere, a record of it was sought. All hospitalizations were recorded. The parents were assured that the green discharge card was a passport to prompt medical treatment in our hospital.

The development of the child was first assessed by the neonatologist and occupational therapist by the Amiel-Tison and occupational therapist's method **(Annexure II)**. The infant was sent for testing with the Bayley Scales of Infant Development at 3, 6, 9, and 12 months, since Dr Pramila Phatak had not developed the Developmental Assessment Scales for Indian Infants (DASII) test till 1996. Corrected age was used in preterms. Raval's scale of social maturity was also used. This scale is particularly useful in children with cerebral palsy.

Therefore, 425 consecutive babies discharged from the NICU were identified by predetermined criteria. 161 infants (37.9%) were full term, out of which 54.6% were small for gestational age (SGA) **(Table 1)**. Out of the 264 preterm infants, 57.9% were SGA. Out of the 404 babies who could be traced, 38 (9.4%) died in the first year. The mortality of the babies who did not attend the HRC was 27.6%, compared to those who attended HRC regularly (6.4%), a statistically significant difference.

Most of the families preferred to get admitted to our pediatric ward. Many a times, if they were admitted elsewhere, they requested a transfer to our hospital. A total number of 95 (22.5%) babies had 114 admissions to the hospital, out of these 87 were admitted in the first year of life.

Thus, 336 babies came for regular follow-ups. The neurologic sequelae are shown in **Table 2**.

264 preterm infants with gestation <37 weeks were discharged from our unit during the study period. Out of these preterm infants, only those who had at least two testings in the first 12 months and at least one subsequent testing before 24 months were included. Almost 172 infants fulfilled these criteria. **Table 2** shows the birth weight and gestational age of these infants. Infants who had an uneventful course in the NICU and had no risk factors other than prematurity and low birth weight (LBW) were called "uncomplicated" preterms. 63 infants were uncomplicated and 109 (63.3%) infants had other risk factors. The "uncomplicated" preterms had mental and motor quotients in the nineties and caught up with controls between 12 and 18 months. Whereas

TABLE 1: Birth weight and gestation of high-risk infants.

Birth weight (g)	n	%	Gestation (weeks)	n	%
≥2,500	58	17.3	≥37	128	38.0
2,001–2,499	29	8.6	35–36	84	25.2
1,751–2,000	44	13.0	33–34	81	24.2
1,501–1,750	93	27.6	31–32	36	10.7
1,251–1,500	73	21.6	29–30	6	1.7
1,001–1,250	33	09.8	≤28	1	0.2
≥1,000	6	1.7	–	–	–
Total	336			336	

TABLE 2: Neurologic sequelae in 336 high-risk infants (Preterm—208, LBW—258, VLBW—109).

Sequelae	n	%
Cerebral palsy:	16	4.8
• Spastic quadriplegia	8	2.4
• Athetoid	4	1.2
• Spastic diplegia	2	0.6
• Hemiplegia	2	0.6
Mental retardation:	17	5.0
• With cerebral palsy	11	3.3
• Without cerebral palsy	6	1.8
Seizure disorders:	13	3.9
• Generalized	9	2.1
• Focal	1	0.3
• Infantile myoclonus	3	0.9
Hearing impairment:	5	1.5
• Sensorineural deafness	4	1.2
• Only high frequency loss	1	0.3
Cortical blindness	1	0.3

(LBW: low birth weight; VLBW: very low birth weight)

TABLE 3: Neurological assessment at 3 months and outcome at 12 months (n = 111).

3-month examination	12 months	Outcome
	Major neuromotor abnormality	Normal
Abnormal (n = 45)	12	33
Normal (n = 66)	2	64

the infants with additional risk factors had much lower quotients and caught up with controls between 18 and 24 months. The preterm appropriate for gestational age (AGA) babies caught up with controls at 18 months.[1] But the babies who were SGA, took longer and caught up with controls at 24 months.

Out of the 172 preterm infants in this study, 7 (4.1%) had frank cerebral palsy with 3 having associated mental retardation. 4 infants (2.3%) had severe mental retardation.[2] The prospects for development of these preterm infants appeared bright, if they were appropriate for gestational age and had no other complications.

111 babies who had a 3-month testing and a 12-month testing with the Amiel-Tison method were analyzed to see if the 3-month testing could predict normality at 12 months **(Table 3)**. The predictive value for a negative test (normality) was 96.9%. This indicates that if the neurological assessment was normal at 3 months, the chances are that the baby will have normal motor development at 12 months.[3]

REFERENCES

1. Chaudhari S, Kulkarni S, Pajnigar, Pandit AN, Deshmukh S. A longitudinal follow up of development of preterm infants. Indian Pediatr. 1991;28(8):873-80.
2. Chaudhari S, Kulkarni S, Barve S, Pandit AN, Sonak U, Sarpotdar N. Neurologic sequelae in high risk infants: A three-year follow-up. Indian Pediatr. 1996;33(8):645-53.
3. Chaudhari S, Kulkarni S, Barve S, Pandit A. Neurological assessment at 3 months as a predictor for development in high risk infants. Indian Pediatr. 1993;30(4):528-31.

PHASE II

An In-depth Longitudinal Study of Development in High-risk Infants from 5 to 6 Years

Stanford–Binet Test

The children were now of school-going age and needed more exhaustive assessment of their intellect. Intelligence quotient (IQ) was done using the Stanford–Binet test which has an Indian adaptation by Kulshrestha. The mean IQ of the high-risk children (96.12 ± 14.06) was significantly lower than that of controls (104.6 ± 12.1) **(Table 4)**.

Children with borderline intelligence were identified (IQ 70–84). Among the 286 high-risk children, 42 (14.68) were in this group.[1]

A school visit was done and an interview with the teacher using Connor's teacher rating scale was attempted, to find out the behavior in school of these children. However, this interview was not very informative. Many teachers said that there were 60 children in the class and it was impossible for them

TABLE 4: Comparison of mean intelligence quotients (IQs) of controls with study group at 12 years.

Group	n	Mean IQ (SD)	p value
Controls	71	101.38 (10.2)	--
All LBW	201	94.30 (13.6)	0.000
Full-term SGA	35	96.02 (15.4)	0.03
Preterm AGA	79	95.85 (14.6)	0.009
Preterm SGA	87	92.22 (11.6)	0.000

(AGA: appropriate for gestational age; SD: standard deviation; LBW: low birth weight; SGA: small for gestational age)

to answer such probing questions. Some teachers got irritated and answered in the negative for all questions. So this effort was quite unrewarding, as the teachers were not cooperative. **Table 4** shows the distribution of IQ at 6 years. We asked the children to get their school reports at the end of the year. There was good correlation between the school performance and IQ.

Bender–Gestalt Test

This test was done to assess visuomotor perception. The number of children who performed this test was much smaller because many of them did not complete the test of nine pictures, and some lost interest after the long IQ test. But the visuomotor perception was much poorer in high-risk children.

Draw a Man Test (Phatak)

Human figure drawing (Koppitz): Human figure drawing on a specified piece of paper was analyzed to give IQ and emotional indicators. The difference between emotional indicators of high-risk and control children was not significant.

Occupational Therapy (Ayres)

This assessment was done by the therapist in the following headings:
- Gross motor activity
- Fine motor activity
- Perception
- Language
- Preschool skills
- Activities of daily living (ADL)

The number of high-risk children needing assistance was significantly higher for language development. Similarly, the number of children with abnormal preschool skills was significantly higher than controls.

Social and Environmental Factors[2]

The impact of social and environment factors cannot be overlooked. A regression analysis showed that mother's education and spaciousness of the house were two important factors influencing the IQ.

Interventions

No assessment is meaningful unless appropriate intervention is offered.

Medical Intervention

The main role of the physician was to act as a liaison officer, other than managing routine medical problems. He gave advice regarding immunization, especially for some of the newer vaccines. He coerced parents of children with "borderline intelligence" to change from an English medium school to a Marathi medium school. He also explained the importance of the occupational therapist's intervention.

Psychologist's Intervention

The psychologist's intervention was done for children with behavior problems, attention deficit disorders, emotional disturbances, and scholastic problems. They used play therapy and behavior modification therapy. They also advised special methods of teaching and stimulation in children with borderline intelligence.

Occupational Therapy Intervention[3]

When children were found to have problems in gross and fine motor activities, intersensory integration, preschool skills, and ADL, they were given a home-based program if the problems were mild. When the problems were severe, they were called to our in-house TDH rehabilitation centre for therapy.

Audiology Intervention

Six children were given hearing aids and special training was given to parents. Speech training was given to one child who had mild hearing loss. Parents of two children received financial support from voluntary organizations for buying hearing aids. Six children with dyslalia were given few sessions of speech therapy, and parents were taught how to talk with these children.

Ophthalmology Intervention

Children with refractive errors were given glasses. One child had a cataract and was operated and an intraocular implant was put. Three children with squint were advised surgery. Three children with squint had hypermetropia and were given corrective glasses.

Mortality and Morbidity during a 6-year Follow-up

There were 40 deaths during the 6-year follow-up, out of which 38 deaths occurred during the first year, 22 in the hospital and 16 at home. About 60% of these deaths were in the first 3 months, and 72% of the deaths were due to infection.

The mortality in the very low birth weight (VLBW) group was significantly higher than the rest of the group. There was a trend towards higher mortality in lower socioeconomic group. The mortality amongst the group who attended the High Risk Clinic regularly was significantly lower (6.4%) than that of the defaulters (27.6%).

A total number of 95 children had 144 admissions to the hospital, 87 (91.5%) were admitted in the first year of life. And 35 infants were admitted for infections (gastroenteritis–24, pneumonitis–6, and septicemia–5). Similarly, 20 children were admitted for seizures, 2 for shunt surgery, 8 with protracted diarrhea, and 8 for failure to thrive. Thus 14 infants needed a top-up transfusion for anemia.[4]

The mean IQ of the high-risk group was 98.21 ± 6.2, which was significantly lower than that of controls (101.538 ± 10.2). A significantly larger proportion of high-risk children had "borderline intelligence" (14.7%) as compared to that of controls (5.6%). It was observed that the trend for borderline intelligence increased significantly with decreasing gestation and birth weight.

The IQ of children, who had transient tone abnormalities in the first year by the Amiel-Tison test, was determined at 5 years.[5] These children had normal IQ at 5 years, unlike poor cognitive outcome in these children described by Amiel-Tison.

REFERENCES

1. Chaudhari S, Bhalerao MR, Chitale A, Pandit A, Nene U. Pune low birth weight study: a six year follow up. Indian Pediatr. 1999;36(7):669-76.
2. Kuppuswamy B. Manual of Socio-economic Status Scale. New Delhi: Manayasan Revision; 1991.
3. Hopkins HL, Smith HD. Therapeutic application of activity. In: Hopkins H, Smith H, (Eds). Willard and Packman's Occupational Therapy, 6th edition. Philadelphia: JB Lippincott CO; 1983.pp. 223-30.
4. Chaudhari S, Kulkarni S, Pandit A, Deshmukh S. Mortality and morbidity in high risk infants during a six year follow up. Indian Pediatr. 2000;37(12):1314-20.
5. Chaudhari S, Bhalerao MR, Chitale A, Pandit A, Nene U. Transient tone abnormalities in high risk infants and cognitive outcome at five years. Indian Pediatr. 2010;47(11):931-5.

PHASE III

Growth and Cognitive Development in Low Birth Newborns at 12 years

Nearly one-third of neonates born in India are LBW and a large percentage of them are small for gestational age (SGA). This longitudinal study aims to find out the growth, sexual maturation, and cognitive development of LBW children at 12 years. Comparison between the LBW children and controls is shown in **Table 5**.

The preterm SGA males were lighter, shorter, and had smaller heads compared to controls. Preterm females were shorter, had smaller heads, but were heavier as far as weight was concerned. The full-term SGA children had smaller heads but were comparable in weight and height with controls. There was no difference in sexual maturity in all the groups of both sexes. As this was a prospective study, growth parameters were available since birth and a growth trajectory could be drawn. Preterm SGA children remained short

TABLE 5: Birth data of infants, height, weight, and sociodemographic data of parents.

	PTSGA (n = 73)	FTSGA (n = 33)	PTAGA (n = 74)	Controls (n = 90)
Birth characteristics				
Male : Female	39:34	18:15	45:29	55:35
Mean (SD) birth weight (g)	1419.9 (244.2)	1700.7 (226.9)	1609.2 (178.4)	2853.7 (321.0)
Mean birth weight Z score	−2.6	−3.9	−1.4	−1.4
Mean gestation (SD) (week)	34.4 (1.9)	FT	33.3 (1.3)	FT
Mother's mean height (SD) (cm)	153.5 (7.8)	153.7 (6.4)	154.0 (7.0)	155.3 (6.2)
Father's mean height (SD) (cm)	163.6 (6.1)	165.9 (6.3)	164.7 (6.3)	165.5 (5.7)
Mother's mean weight (SD) (kg)	45.3 (8.7)	45.1 (4.9)	48.0 (11.2)	48.8 (8.9)
Father's mean weight (SD) (kg)	56.6 (10.6)	55.3 (7.1)	60.2 (10.1)	60.0 (9.1)
Socioeconomic status (n%)				
Higher	10 (13.7)	8 (24.2)	15 (20.3)	12 (13.3)
Upper middle	18 (24.7)	6 (18.2)	23 (31.1)	25 (27.8)
Lower middle	27 (37)	14 (42.4)	24 (32.4)	37 (41.1)
Lower	18 (24.7)	5 (15.2)	12 (16.2)	16 (17.8)
Educational status of mother				
<10th Std	31 (42.5%)	12 (36.4%)	30 (40.5%)	33 (36.7%)
≥10th Std	42 (57.5%)	21 (63.6%)	44 (59.5%)	57 (63.3%)

throughout the 12 years, although some "catch up" did occur between 4 and 12 years. Full-term SGA children had the lowest birth weight, Z Score (−3.93), but showed some catch up between 4 and 12 years.[1] All four measurements for adiposity showed that none of the LBW children were in the obese range.

A bone age was determined by taking X-rays of both hands by the method described by Tanner and a prediction of final height was done. The radiologist was blinded to the present height.

The cognitive development was assessed by the following tests mentioned here.

Weschler's Intelligence Scale (WISC-R)

The mean intelligence quotients of LBW and controls are compared in **Table 6**. The verbal IQ was poor in the entire LBW group. The preterm SGA group had the poorest IQ (85.4 ± 177). The preterm appropriate for gestational age (AGA) and full-term SGA group performed better and had IQs in the nineties. The 78 VLBW children performed poorly, with more children with intellectual disability (IQ < 70) and just 3 bright children **(Table 6)**.

Bender–Gestalt Test

Half the LBW children had poor visuomotor perception with visuomotor age <9 years.

TABLE 6: Distribution of IQ (WISC-R) at 12 years.

Intelligence quotient	Study group (n = 180) n (%)	Controls (n = 90) n (%)
50–69 (Retarded)	24 (13.3)**	3 (3.3)
70–84 (Borderline)	44 (24.4)	14 (15.6)
85–109 (Normal)	93 (51.8)	53 (58.9)
>110 (Bright)	19 (10.5)**	20 (22.2)

(IQ: intelligence quotient; WISC-R: Wechsler Intelligence Scale for Children-Revised)
**$p<0.001$

TABLE 7: Comparison of mathematics score (WRAT).

Group	n	Mathematics score mean (SD)
All LBW	180	82.7 (16.9)*
Birthweight <1,500 g	78	80.4 (15.1)**
Birthweight 1,500–1,999 g	102	84.4 (17.9)
Preterm SGA	73	81.6 (18.0)*
Full term SGA	33	82.7 (16.2)
Preterm AGA	74	83.7 (16.1)
Controls	90	87.8 (15.8)

(AGA: appropriate for gestational age; LBW: low birth weight; SGA: small for gestational age; WRAT: Wide Range of Achievement Test)
*$p<0.01$, **$p<0.001$

Wide Range Achievement Test (WRAT)

This test determines reading, writing, and mathematics skills. The reading skills did not show any difference in the LBW and control groups. The writing skills were much poorer in the LBW group. The VLBW children and children with gestation <32 weeks had greater difficulty in writing. The mathematics score of the LBW group (82.7±16.9) was significantly less than that of the controls (87.8 ±15.8). The VLBW and preterm SGA children had very poor scores in mathematics **(Table 7)**.

Movement Assessment Battery (ABC)

This test assesses three motor skills: body balance, ball skills, and manual dexterity. The girls performed poorly in body balance and ball skills but did better in manual dexterity compared to boys. On the whole, the LBW group performed poorly compared to controls.

School Performance

Most of the children were studying in the 7th standard. Amongst the LBW group, seven children gave a history of repeating a grade. There was a strong correlation between school performance and IQ.

Biology versus Environment

In the last century, the primary emphasis in outcome studies was on incidence of major disabilities. While biologic factors are more predictive of major handicaps, social and environmental factors are more predictive of school age outcome in "nonhandicapped" children. Low birth weight children are exposed to a "double jeopardy" of biologic and environmental risks.[2]

Sociodemography

A detailed sociodemographic and environmental background of each child was obtained and confirmed by a home visit by the social worker.

Mother's and father's education: This was divided in four categories: (1) Illiterate, (2) middle school, (3) high school, and (4) college.

Socioeconomic status: This was determined by using the revised Kuppuswamy scale and divided into four categories: (1) Lower class, (2) lower middle class, (3) upper middle class, and (4) upper class. The family size was determined by the number of people living in the same house: (1) >10 persons, (2) 6-10 persons, and (3) <5 persons. A note was made if a single parent was bringing up the child.

Spaciousness of the house: It was calculated by the number of persons sharing a room: (1) more than 3 persons, (2) 3 persons, and (3) 1-2 persons.

School: The school attended by the child was classified into three categories: (1) Municipal corporation school, (2) average school, and (3) good school.

Locality: The locality in which the child lived was divided in four categories: (1) Slums, (2) lower middle, (3) upper middle, and (4) high class.

Breastfeeding

We recorded the age upto which exclusive breastfeeding was done.

Stimulation and Parenting

The stimulation received by the child at home, the "care giving environment" at different ages was assessed using different tests. The initial assessment was done at 6 and 12 months to determine early stimulation. An interaction score was calculated at 3 years.

Family Environment Scale

This scale was used at 12 years. This scale consisted of three main divisions: (1) Relationship dimensions, (2) personal growth dimensions, and (3) system maintenance dimensions.

Cognitive Assessment[3]

This was assessed by a trained psychologist using Weschler's Intelligence Scale (WISCR) and Wide Range Achievement Test (WRAT).

Children who had mothers with college education had far superior IQs than children whose mothers had lesser education. Similar findings were seen

TABLE 8: Determinants of intelligence quotient (IQ)—multiple linear regression analysis.

Dependent variable	Independent variable	Beta	Adjusted R^2	Total variance (%)	Contribution to total variance (%)
Total IQ				44.2	
	Mother's education	0.290	0.252		25.2
	School	0.284	0.338		8.6
	Birth weight	0.213	0.379		4.1
	Spaciousness	0.167	0.405		2.6
	FES—expressiveness	0.145	0.426		2.1
	FES—control	−0.141	0.442		1.6
Performance IQ				32.4	
	Mother's education	0.294	0.176		17.6
	Birth weight	0.231	0.239		6.3
	School	0.245	0.275		3.6
	FES-control	−0.183	0.304		2.9
Verbal IQ				34.6	
	School	0.321	0.220		22
	Father's education	0.190	0.297		7.7
	3-year stimulation score	0.196	0.325		2.8
	FES—expressiveness	0.167	0.346		2.1
Mathematics score				36.4	
	Father's education	0.360	0.256		25.6
	School	0.320	0.342		8.6
	FES—control	0.166	0.364		2.2

(FES: family environmental scale; IQ: intelligence quotient)

with father's education. The stimulation score did not show any significant difference between the two groups.[2]

Thus, the cognitive development of "non-handicapped" LBW children depended mainly on mother's education, father's education, and the type of school attended by the child. Birth weight was the only biologic factor, which had a small contribution to later IQ **(Table 8)**.

REFERENCES

1. Chaudhari S, Otiv M, Hoge M, Pandit A, Mote A. Growth and sexual maturation of low birth weight infants at early adolescence. Indian Pediatr. 2008;45(3):191-8.
2. Chaudhari S, Otiv M, Chitale A, Hoge M, Pandit A, Mote A. Biology versus environment in low birth weight children. Indian Pediatr. 2005;42(8):763-70.
3. Chaudhari S, Otiv M, Chitale A, Pandit A, Hoge M. Pune low birth weight study: cognitive abilities and educational performance at twelve years. Indian Pediatr. 2004;41(2):121-8.

PHASE IV

Pune Low Birth Weight Study: Birth to Adulthood

The LBW children whom we had been following since birth had reached adulthood. So we decided to assess their final growth, and their final IQ.

Since the children had cooperated with us for such a long follow-up, we felt that we should give them something in return. So we did an aptitude test so that we could give them career guidance. We now know from Professor Barker's studies that children who had suffered intrauterine growth restriction were more likely to develop the "metabolic syndrome". Hence we took detailed measurements for adiposity.

At 18 years, 161 LBW young adults and 73 controls were available for follow-up, with great effort. We had managed to get 80% of our original cohort. Out of the 131 preterms, 61% were small for gestational age (SGA). There were 71 VLBW infants.

Assessments of Growth

The preterm SGA (PTSGA) males were the shortest in the group, the PTSGA females did not show a significant difference in height compared to control females. PTSGA females had a significantly smaller head compared to control females. VLBW subjects were significantly shorter and had smaller heads.[1]

We had done a bone age of all LBW children at 12 years and the radiologist had predicted their final height. The actual height at 18 years was strongly in agreement with the predicted height. A multiple regression analysis was done to look for determinant of height, weight, and head circumference. Mother's and father's height were important determinants for height, mother's and father's weight were important determinants for weight and birth weight and gender were determinants of head circumference.

When we compared measurements for adiposity [body mass index (BMI), waist and hip circumference, waist/height ratio and sum of four skin-fold thicknesses], there was no difference between the LBW group and controls.

Assessments of Cognition

Raven's Progressive Matrices

This is a performance test of intelligence. It evaluates the subject's ability to apprehend relationships, geometric figures, and designs and to perceive the structure of design in order to select the appropriate part. It is a test of innate educational ability with a small contribution of spatial perception factor.

The IQ of the LBW group was significantly lower than that of controls.[2] The PTSGA had significantly more subjects with IQ below average compared to controls. Preterm appropriate for gestational age (AGA) subjects had lower IQ than controls but still within normal limits. VLBW subjects had significantly low IQ. School failures were higher in the study group. Failures were more in boys compared to girls. Preterm SGA children of college-educated mothers had far better IQs compared to those with mothers with lesser education.

In order to find out at what age we could predict the 18-year IQ, we did a correlation with the MDI at 1 year, IQ at 6, and 12 years. The best correlation was seen with the 6- and 12-year IQ.

Assessments of Adjustment

The adjustment inventory taps the relationship between the individual and his environment in five areas:
1. Family environment
2. Social adjustment
3. Personal and emotional adjustment
4. Education adjustment
5. Health adjustment

We found no difference in the adjustment between the subjects and controls and also between boys and girls.

Assessments of Aptitude

This was done by the differential aptitude test which tests the following abilities:
- Numerical ability
- Abstract reasoning
- Space relations
- Mechanical reasoning
- Clerical speed and accuracy

Those subjects with aptitude for space relations opted for fine arts. Those who were poor in speed opted for arts colleges. Those who had poor abstract thinking and mechanical reasoning opted for commerce.

This study may not be relevant for tertiary care units, who are saving ELBW babies today. However, there are many Level II care units in India, especially in smaller towns. The methodology of this study and the tests used for determining various aspects of development at different ages may serve as a model for planning future follow-up studies of ELBW infants.

REFERENCES

1. Chaudhari S, Otiv M, Khairnar B, Pandit A, Hoge M, Sayyad M. Pune low birth weight study—growth from birth to adulthood. Indian Pediatr. 2012;49(9):727-32.
2. Chaudhari S, Otiv M, Khairnar B, Pandit N, Hoge M, Sayyad M. Pune low birth weight study—birth to adulthood: cognitive development. Indian Pediatr. 2013;50(9):853-7.

PHASE V

Prevalence of Markers of "Metabolic Syndrome" in a Cohort of Low Birth Weight Children at Early Adulthood

India is experiencing an epidemic of type II diabetes and coronary heart disease in young adults and middle-aged population. The World Health Organization has projected a 300% rise in deaths due to cardiovascular (CHD) disease in 2025 in India, as opposed to a rise of 40% in the Western countries. Epidemiologic studies have shown a strong correlation between small size at birth and increased risk for CHD and type II diabetes. The cluster of risk factors of CHD, type II diabetes, hypertension, dyslipidemia, and abdominal obesity is known as "metabolic syndrome." The Barker hypothesis, also known as "fetal origins hypothesis" states that CHD and type II diabetes originated through the adaptations that the fetus makes, when it is undernourished. Since 60% of our LBW cohort was small for gestational age, we thought that this was an ideal cohort to see if we could identify early predictors of "metabolic syndrome".

We recalled our subjects at 22 years to study the parameters of metabolic syndrome (Met-S). The subjects were reluctant to come to the hospital since many of them were working, some were studying in colleges. And 17 girls were married and 4 even had young babies. We offered a free check-up along with blood tests to both their parents and this gesture paid off. Thus, 153 LBW subjects and 77 controls were available for the 22-year follow-up.

The LBW subjects and parents were first examined by the doctor. History of any major illness was recorded. Both parents were asked history of diabetes or hypertension. A physical examination was done. Blood pressure was recorded. Then blood was drawn after an overnight fast for:
- Oral glucose tolerance test
- Lipid profile
- Hemogram

All measurements for adiposity were taken. Height, weight, sitting height, waist circumference, hip circumference, waist hip ratio, mid-arm circumference, and skinfold thickness were measured at four sites (biceps, triceps, subscapular, and suprailiac). A body mass index (BMI) and sum of four skinfold thickness was calculated. The height and sitting height differed significantly between male cases and controls. Amongst the females, the sitting height and biceps skinfold thickness differed significantly between cases and controls.

The diastolic blood pressure was significantly higher in male and female subjects. All the mean biochemical parameters such as fasting, 30 minute, 120 minute blood sugars, total and high-density lipoprotein (HDL) cholesterol, and triglycerides were within normal limits. We then compared the components of Met-S between the LBW group and controls (2001 NCEP–ATP guidelines).
- Waist circumference >102 cm in men and >88 cm in women was found in nine cases and two controls.
- Serum triglycerides $\geq$150 mg/dL (1.7 mmol/L) were seen in 13 cases and 4 controls.
- Fasting glucose >110 mg/dL (6.1 mmol/L was seen in three cases and no controls).
- HDL $\leq$40 mg/dL (1.03 mmol/L) and <50 mg (1.229 mmol/L) in women was seen in 109 cases and 55 controls.
- The presence in three components of Met-S was seen in only three cases and no controls. However, presence of two components of Met-S was seen in 25 cases (16.4%), as opposed to only 5 controls, a significant difference.

A magnetic resonance imaging (MRI) of abdomen was done to measure subcutaneous fat in the abdominal wall. There was no significant difference in the subcutaneous fat between cases and controls. An ultrasonography was done on 3rd to 5th day of menstruation to look for polycystic ovarian syndrome (PCOD), but only six girls had PCOD.

We were fortunate to have a dietician in our project. She took a detailed dietetic history (week days and week end) by 24 hours diet recall and physical activity was assessed by using a questionnaire. Since the mothers were present, the dietician gave advice regarding proper diet. She also advised them regarding physical activity.

Insulin levels were measured and insulin resistance (Home-IR) was calculated. A multiple regression analysis showed that sum of four skinfold thickness was a significant determinant of HOMA-IR. Similarly, sum of four skinfold thickness was a significant determinant of 120-minute blood glucose. So taking this measurement in young LBW adults is very important.

Higher BMI at 2, 6, 12, and 18 years correlated significantly with higher blood pressure. Higher BMI at 12 years correlated significantly with higher fasting insulin and higher HOMA-IR at 22 years.

The birth weight and 22-year weight was divided in four quartiles. Those who were born small and remained small at 22 years were compared with those who were born small, but became big at 22 years. Fasting, 30-minute, 120-minute insulin, and HOMA-IR were significantly higher in those born small and became big at 22 years. Serum cholesterol and triglycerides were higher, blood pressure was higher and abdominal obesity on MRI was more in this group.

When the BMI of parents was compared separately with that of cases, the BMI of parents correlated with BMI of cases. When the incidence of the components of Met-S between those having family history of diabetes and cardiovascular disease, and those not having family history was compared, there was no significant difference. During our study, six parents were found to be pre-diabetic, two were frank diabetic, five parents had hypertension and none of them were aware of it.

These 25 cases, who are showing two components of Met-S, may be heading for a frank Met-S 10 years from now. Since this was a research project with an inbuilt therapeutic program, advice regarding change in the lifestyle was given.

BIBLIOGRAPHY

1. Chaudhari S, Otiv, Hoge M, Pandit A, Sayyed M. Components of metabolic syndrome at 22 years of age: findings from Pune low birth weight study. Indian Pediatr. 2017;54(6):461-7.

Pune Neurodevelopmental Screening Test

CHAPTER 12

Sudha Chaudhari

INTRODUCTION

This test was devised as a quick screening test for high-risk infants in a busy office practice. With our vast experience of testing high-risk babies with the Amiel-Tison (AT) method[1] and the Development Assessment Scale for Indian Infants (DASII),[2] we took some salient features of both the tests and devised a simple testing kit. 125 infants were tested at 3, 6, 9, and 12 months cross-sectionally. Corrected age was used in preterms. They were first assessed by the AT method and then by the DASII method. A sensitivity and specificity was calculated. This test is not published.

Cochrane and Holland have described six criteria for a screening test: (1) It should be simple, quick, and easy to interpret, (2) acceptable, in order to encourage participation in a screening program, (3) accurate, to give true measurement under investigation, (4) repeatable, (5) sensitive, and (6) specific.

The Pune neurodevelopmental screening test fulfilled all these criteria.

A simple inexpensive kit was put together: (1) A small red ball for visual fixation and pursuit, (2) a "pooja" bell for testing hearing at 3 months, (3) a piece of paper used for crackling, to test hearing 6 months onward, (4) a red pen and rattle for testing handedness and transfer, (5) a colored paper clip for testing pincer grasp, (6) a paper and a pen for scribbling either imitative or spontaneous at 12 months, and (7) a tape measure. The cost of the whole kit was Rs. 50 **(Fig. 1)**. The whole test takes 5–7 minutes.

Here are few suggestions while doing the test: Do not ask the mother to put the baby on the examining table. Pick up the baby yourself and put him/her on the table. You are inadvertently doing the axillary suspension maneuver. If the baby is hypotonic, he will slip from your hands, if he is hypertonic, he may scissor. When the baby is 6 months or older and you are talking to the mother, put a couple of toys in front of the baby on the table. The baby should not show any handedness. If the baby uses only one hand persistently, look out for hemiparesis which may have been missed. Crackle a piece of paper outside the visual field of the baby. If the baby hears this sound, he will turn toward the sound.

This test does not replace the other neurodevelopmental tests. This is the first step, a simple screening test.

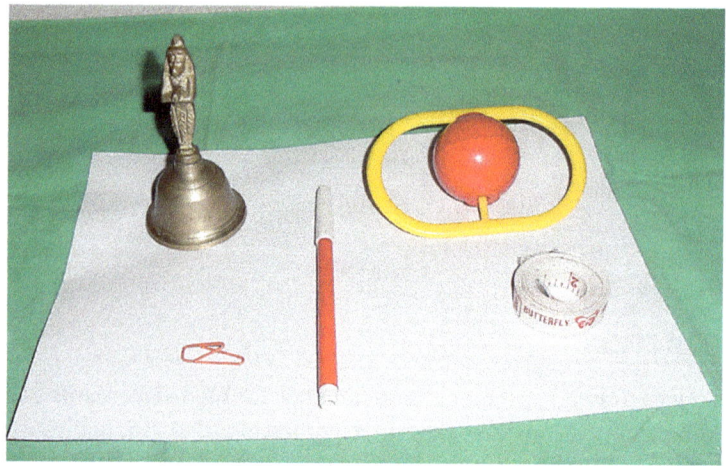

Fig. 1: Simple neurodevelopmental screening test kit.

NEUROLOGICAL EXAMINATION OF NEWBORNS AND INFANTS IN OFFICE PRACTICE

3 months

1. History for neurobehavior : Cry, lethargy/irritability
   Feeding problems
   Seizures, sleep pattern
   Response to sound, light
   Social smile
2. Head growth : Head circumference
   Anterior fontanelle
   Sutures
3. Eyes : Tone LPS/setting-sun sign
   Strabismus, nystagmus, any other
   Roving eye movements for cortical blindness
4. Neurosensory : Follows red ball
   Turns toward sound
5. Posture and spontaneous activity : Spontaneous asymmetrical tonic neck reflex (ATNR), facial asymmetry
   Hypertonia neck extensors
   Opisthotonus, fisting
6. Passive tone : Adductor angle, scarf sign, dorsiflexion
   Angle of foot (for TA tightness)
7. Active tone : Supports head
8. Axillary suspension : Slips from hands, head/neck control, scissoring

9.	Neonatal reflexes	:	Moro, automatic walking, Palmar grasp to see if reflexes have disappeared
10.	Reflexes [deep tendon reflexes (DTR)]	:	Ankle clonus
11.	Mental milestones	:	Social smile
12.	Stimulation program	:	Prone position (for head control), red ball, bell/rattle, soft music
13.	Therapy	:	If hypertonia—no oil massage If neck extensor hypertonia—"Zoli" or hammock. Do *not* label as abnormal If opisthotonus No head control, no social smile Or any other abnormality—refer to therapist

6 months

1.	History for neurobehavior	:	Feeding problems Seizures Vision Hearing-response to sounds
2.	Head growth	:	Head circumference Anterior fontanelle Sutures
3.	Eyes	:	Tone LPS/setting-sun sign Strabismus, nystagmus
4.	Neurosensory	:	Vision Response to crackling of paper and Pooja bell
5.	Posture and spontaneous activity	:	Symmetrical (Look out for ATNR, opisthotonus, hyper/hypotonia, general fisting, asymmetry)
6.	Passive tone	:	Adductor angle, scarf sign, Dorsiflexion of foot (for TA tightness)
7.	Active tone and milestones	:	Pull-to-sit—no head lag, momentary sitting for 30 sec atleast rolls over, pulls to stand
8.	Axillary suspension	:	Slips through hands Spontaneous scissoring of lower limbs General hypertonia

9. Neonatal reflexes : Check for Moro, should have disappeared
10. Reflexes : Ankle clonus/biceps jerk
11. Mental milestones : Recognizes mother by 4 months
Voluntary reach, transfer of objects
12. Stimulation program : Play with katori and spoon, sit with support in a corner
13. Therapy : If adductor tightness: carrying pattern—astride
If TA tightness or any asymmetry—reference to therapist
If hypotonia—carry with legs together

9 months

1. History for neurobehavior : Seizures
2. Head growth : Head circumference
Anterior fontanelle
Sutures
3. Eyes : Tone LPS/setting-sun sign
Strabismus, nystagmus
4. Neurosensory : Vision, hearing
5. Posture and spontaneous activity : Symmetrical
Look out for any asymmetry
Normal/increased/decreased, ambidextrous
If hand preference—abnormal
6. Axillary suspension : Slips through hands
Spontaneous scissoring of lower limbs
General hypertonia
7. Passive tone : Adductor angle, scarf sign, dorsiflexion of foot angle (for TA tightness)
8. Active tone and milestones : Pull to sit, pulls to stand
Sits alone with straight back
Weight bearing on feet (comes back)
9. Motor milestones : Sits without support
Crawls
Stands with support

10. Mental milestones	:	Discriminates strangers, pincer grasp *Imitative behavior:* • Clap clap • Peek a boo
11. Neonatal reflexes	:	Should have disappeared, lateral propping parachute reflexes
12. Reflexes (Deep tendon reflexes)	:	Ankle clonus
13. Stimulation program	:	Climbing on mother's body for standing
14. Therapy	:	Tone abnormality or developmental delay, OT intervention

12 months

1. History for neurobehavior	:	Seizures Therapy given at any stage
2. Head growth	:	Head circumference Anterior fontanelle Sutures
3. Eyes	:	Any abnormality
4. Neurosensory	:	Vision Hearing
5. Posture and spontaneous activity	:	Look out for any asymmetry General hypertonia, hypotonia
6. Axillary suspension	:	Slips through hands Scissoring Hypertonia—generalized
7. Passive tone	:	Adductor angle, scarf sign, dorsiflexion angle of foot (for TA tightness)
8. Active tone and milestones	:	Pulls to stand
9. Motor milestones	:	Sits without support Walks sideways along furniture (cruising) stands
10. Mental milestones	:	Pincer grasp Responds to his name Rings bell purposefully Says single word Scribbles with pen after demonstration
11. Neonatal reflexes	:	Should have disappeared Parachute reaction (+)

12. Deep tendon reflexes : Biceps/ankle
13. Stimulation program : Showing single picture on single page
14. Therapy : Tone abnormal/developmental delay—refer

REFERENCES

1. Amiel-Tison C. A method for neurological evaluation with first year of life. Current Problems in Pediatrics VII No 1. Chicago: Year Book Medical Publishers. 1976; pp.1-50.
2. Phatak P, Misra N. Developmental assessment scales for Indian infants (DASII) 1–30 months: Revision of Baroda norms with indigenous material. Psychol Stud. 1996;41: 55-6.

CHAPTER 13

A Parents' Perspective

As narrated by the mother to Dr Sudha Chaudhari

I came to Pune to my mother's place for my first delivery, as is customary in Maharashtra. It was a full-term delivery, so I was not worried but really excited at the prospect of becoming a mother. My son was born with the cord round his neck and did not cry immediately after birth. He was transferred to the neonatal intensive care unit (NICU), kept in an incubator, and given oxygen. I was absolutely devastated that I could not be with my baby and could not breastfeed him. After he was discharged, I stayed on in Pune for 3 months and then came to Nashik, where I live.

I was very anxious about his development. He was 9 months old, but not even sitting up or holding his head. I consulted my family doctor and he said that some children do sit late. He was continuously drooling, and not lifting his right arm at all **(Fig. 1)**. I was not satisfied with this answer and decided to go back to Pune. I knew that Pune being a bigger city with several medical colleges, would have better facilities.

My son was seen by a Developmental Pediatrician and I heard the word "cerebral palsy" for the first time in my life. I was told that he would require prolonged therapy to achieve his milestones. I came back to Nashik, started physiotherapy, but that was not enough. Then I thought that one day if he grows up being handicapped and asks me, "Ma, why did you not try hard to make me normal?" I would have no answer. So I decided to move to Pune.

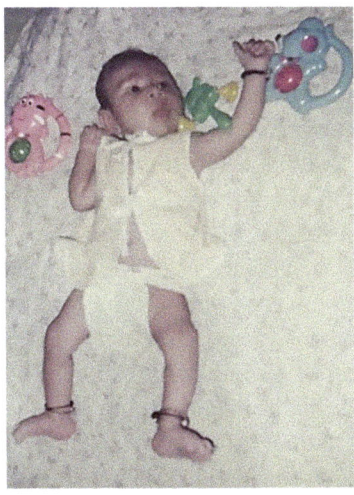

Fig. 1: 9-month-old Rudra unable to raise his right arm.

I started occupational therapy at the TDH Rehabilitation Centre of KEM Hospital, Pune. I was petrified when I saw the various types of children that came to this center for therapy. The diagnosis written on my case paper was "Spastic Quadriplegia with more involvement of the right side." The head of the Occupational Therapy Unit told me two things: (1) I had to have faith in the therapist and follow her instructions assiduously, and (2) The keyword was "patience," since this was going to be a long drawn-out process.

We started going to the center in the morning, and we did the exercises at home in the evening, with the help of my mother. He used to scream during the exercises, probably because they were painful as he was very stiff (spastic). I used to be reduced to tears seeing his pain, but I carried on with unrelenting resolve.

It took 6 months before I saw any signs of improvement. He started sitting up with great effort, started raising his arm a little. I used to bombard the therapists with doubts and queries, and they would utter only two words, "have patience." My father was a pillar of support during these difficult times. My husband also went through hard times, since he could visit us only during weekends, since Nashik is 5 hours away.

He had a developmental assessment (DASII), and was found to have a borderline developmental quotient (DQ). At 30 months, we started speech therapy at the center and his speech started improving slowly. He continued to have a lot of spasticity. At the age of 2 and a half years, it was suggested that he should have Botox treatment. I thought only actresses took Botox injections to enhance their beauty! I was told that he will have plaster on his legs for 15–20 days, and this will have to be followed by intensive therapy and exercises. The effect of the Botox injection would last for 8–9 months and this would give a window to the therapist to strengthen the spastic muscles **(Fig. 2)**.

All this therapy would not have been possible without strong family support. I stayed with my parents for 8 years. Initially, my husband was not happy with this arrangement. But once he saw the gradual progress our son was making, he came round. He made special peg boards to improve his hand function, special shoes [ankle foot orthosis (AFO)], which we kept on during the whole day. He made a special cerebral palsy (CP) chair for him. To improve his fine motor activities, I made him knead dough, shell peas, and peel oranges. Sometimes I would get really dejected, then my husband would give me moral support. Other than occupational and speech therapy, the various workshops taken for parents by the staff of TDH and the guest speakers from Mumbai, really boosted our morale and gave us courage and hope. When he took his first independent step at the age of 4 years, our joy knew no bounds.

We both like to go hiking, so we used to take him with us to climb small hills. At the age of 15 years, he climbed the Kalsubai peak, the highest peak in Maharashtra **(Fig. 3)**. He has a slight limp, but manages to walk well. He likes to dance and performs in dance programs in school. In fact, he performed a dance at the 40 year celebration of the TDH Centre recently. He is now 16 years old and studying in Std X. He has a "borderline" intelligence quotient (IQ), likes

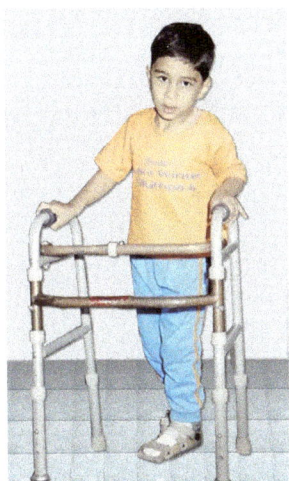 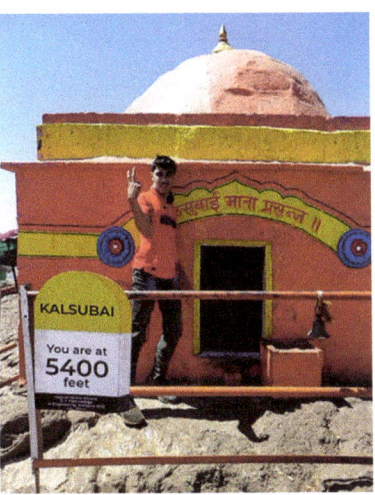

Fig. 2: After Botox injection at the age of 3 years.

Fig. 3: Climbed the highest peak in Maharashtra.

mathematics, physics, and chemistry. He does not like descriptive subjects such as languages, because it involves a lot of writing. He has a cheerful and smiley disposition, and all the hardships. I went through seem unimportant, when I see his progress.

Annexures

- **Annexure I:** Neurological Assessment in the First Year
- **Annexure II:** Combined Neurological Assessment of Neonatologist and Occupational Therapist
- **Annexure III:** High-Risk Follow-up Clinic: Neurological Assessment
- **Annexure IV:** Stimulation Program for Infants

Neurological Assessment in the First Year

ANNEXURE

Name .... Sex ....
Registration No ....
Date of Birth .... Corrected Date ....

(Tick in the appropriate square)

HEAD CIRCUMFERENCE

Months	1	2	3	4	5	6	7	8	9	10	11	12
cm												
SD												

ANTERIOR FONTANELLE

Normal												
Tense												

SUTURES

Normal												
Separated												

PATTERN FOR WAKEFULNESS AND SLEEP

Normal												
Agitated, too much crying												
Lethargic, no crying												

CRY

Normal												
High-pitched												
Weak												

CONVULSIONS DURING THE PRECEDING MONTH

Generalized
Focal
Infantile spasms

| | 1 | 2 | 3 | 4 | 5 | 6 | 7 | 8 | 9 | 10 | 11 | 12 |

SETTING-SUN SIGN

| | 1 | 2 | 3 | 4 | 5 | 6 | 7 | 8 | 9 | 10 | 11 | 12 |
Present

MARKED STRABISMUS

Present

SUSTAINED NYSTAGMUS

Present

PURSUIT OF LIGHT

Present
Absent

RESPONSE TO "POOJA" BELL

Present
Absent

ASYMMETRIC TONIC NECK REFLEX

Absent
Present

HYPERTONICITY OF NECK EXTENSORS

Present

OPISTHOTONOS

Present

FISTING

Present

SPONTANEOUS MOTOR ACTIVITY

Low
Normal
High
Asymmetric

	1	2	3	4	5	6	7	8	9	10	11	12

ABNORMAL MOVEMENTS

	1	2	3	4	5	6	7	8	9	10	11	12
Incessant tremor												
Clonic movements												

ADDUCTOR ANGLE

Angles Mean SD	70–94° *84.8 (6.5)	90–112° *103.8 (8.0)	101–125° *114.1 (6.2)	118–142° *126.6 (5.3)
Angles				

*Indian norms

POPLITEAL ANGLE

Angles Mean SD	90–100° *100.6 (5.4)	100–122° *115.3 (6.1)	110–132° *123.0 (5.6)	120–144° *136.0 (4.0)
Angles				

*Indian norms

DORSIFLEXION ANGLE

Angles Mean SD	50–59° *55.0 (2.7)	52–64° *57.6 (3.3)	55–68° *62.7 (3.4)	58–72° *65.5 (4.6)
Slow angle				
Rapid angle				
Rapid–slow >10°				

*Indian norms

SCARF SIGN

Normal pattern	Elbow medial to midline	Elbow at midline	Elbow crosses midline (to opposite side)	Elbow crosses midline
	①	②	③	④
Limited				
Exaggerated				

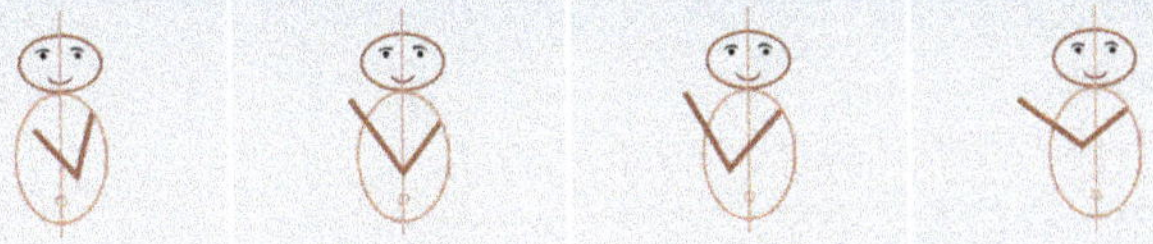

	1	2	3	4	5	6	7	8	9	10	11	12

VENTRAL FLEXION OF THE TRUNK

	1	2	3	4	5	6	7	8	9	10	11	12
Normal (slight)												
Exaggerated												
Impossible												

DORSAL EXTENSION OF THE TRUNK

Normal (slight)	
Exaggerated	

HEAD CONTROL

	Absent	Nonconsistent	present
Normal			
Absent			

PULL-TO-SITTING POSITION

	1	2	3	4	5	6	7	8	9	10	11	12
	Absent				Nonconsistent				Present			
Normal												
Absent												

SITS ALONE MOMENTARILY

	Absent	Nonconsistent	Present
Normal			
Collapses forward			
Falls backward			

SUPPORT REACTION

	Present	Non-consistent	Absent	Possible not sustained	Present
Normal					
Absent					
Scissoring					

MORO REFLEX

	Present	Nonconsistent	Absent
Normal			
Absent			

ANKLE CLONUS

Present

LATERAL PROPPING REACTION

	Absent			Nonconsistent	Present
Present					
Absent					

PARACHUTE

	1	2	3	4	5	6	7	8	9	10	11	12
	Absent			*Absent*			*Nonconsistent*			*Present*		
Present												
Absent												

SUMMARY OF FINDINGS

MICROCEPHALY				
HYDROCEPHALUS				
ABNORMALITIES OF PASSIVE TONE				
ABNORMALITIES OF ACTIVE TONE				
IMPAIRED HEARING				
IMPAIRED VISION				
SQUINT				
DEVELOPMENTAL DELAY				
SEIZURES				
	1–3 months	4–6 months	7–9 months	10–12 months

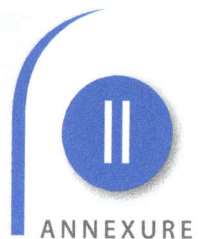

Combined Neurological Assessment of Neonatologist and Occupational Therapist

ANNEXURE

Name: .... Sex: ....
Date of Birth: ..../......../........ Corrected Age:............ HRC No. ....

S. No.	Test	3 months	6 months	9 months	12 months
I. Test					
1.	Head circumference (cm)				
2.	Percentile				
3.	Anterior fontanelle				
4.	Sutures				
5.	Wakefulness and sleep				
6.	Alertness				
7.	Cry				
8.	Sucking behavior				
9.	Convulsion preceding				
10.	Tone LPS				
11.	Setting-sun sign				
12.	Strabismus				
13.	Sustained nystagmus				
14.	Pursuit of light				
15.	Acoustic blink				
16.	Constant closure of hands				
17.	Spontaneous motor activity				
18.	Abnormal movements				
19.	Dyskinetic movements of limbs				
20.	Ventral flexion—Head and Trunk				
21.	Dorsal extension—trunk				
22	Lateral flexion—trunk				
23.	Straightening with neck flexion/extension				
24.	Pulls to sitting position				
25.	Sits alone momentarily				
26.	Sits alone 30 seconds/more				
27.	Straightening with LL and trunk				
28.	Lateral propping reaction				

Contd...

Contd...

S. No.	Test	3 months	6 months	9 months	12 months
II. Tonus Behavior					
1.	Hypertonia				
2.	Tone neck extensor				
3.	Facial asymmetry				
4.	Opisthotonus				
5.	Asymmetrical posture of limb				
6.	Postural tone				
7.	Ankle clonus				
III. Angles					
1.	*Adductor angle (R+L)*	70–94° *84.8 (6.5)	90–112° *103.8 (8.0)	101–125° *114.1 (6.2)	118–142° *126.6 (5.3)
	Limited (R/L)				
	Exaggerated				
2.	*Popliteal angle*	90–100° *100.6 (5.4)	100–122° *115.3 (6.1)	110–132° *123.0 (5.6)	120–144° *136.0 (4.0)
	Limited				
	Exaggerated				
3.	*Dorsiflexion of foot*	50–59° *55.0 (2.7)	52–64° *57.6 (3.3)	55–68° *62.7 (3.4)	58–72° *65.5 (4.6)
	Angle (slow)				
	Angle (rapid)				
	Difference 10″	>10°	>10°	>10°	>10°
	Asymmetry				
4.	*Scarf sign*	Does not cross midline	Up to midline	Crosses midline	Crosses midline
	Limited				
	Exaggerated				
	Asymmetry				
*Indian norms					
IV. Reflexes					
1.	Rooting				
2.	Sucking				
3.	Moro				
4.	Galant				
5.	Cross extension				
6.	Neonatal neck righting				
7.	Placing				

Contd...

Contd...

S. No.	Test	3 months	6 months	9 months	12 months
8.	Neonatal positive support				
9.	Automatic walking				
10.	Asymmetrical tonic neck reflex (ATNR)				
11.	Symmetrical tonic neck reflex (STNR)				
12.	Tonic labyrinthine reflex (TLR)				
13.	Palmar grasp				
14.	Plantar grasp				
15.	Landau test				
16.	Parachute reaction				
17.	Neck righting				
18.	Body righting				
19.	Optical righting				
V. Orthopedics					
1.	Range of motion—UE				
	Range of motion—LE				
	Range of motion—Neck				
2.	Contractures/Deformity				
VI. Adaptive Responses					
1.	Self-consolability				
2.	Spontaneous behavior				
VII. Sensory Motor Integration					
1.	Tactile				
2.	*Visual:*				
	• Eyes open				
	• Pursuit of image				
	• Localization				
	• Tracks to midline				
3.	*Auditory:*				
	• Alerts to noise				
	• Activates to voice				
	• Localizes voice				
4.	*Nasal and feeding function:*				
	• Breathing—nasal/oral				
	• Tongue—midline/deviated				
	• Sucking—spontaneous				
	– Lip closure				
	• Swallowing—sequence with suck				
	Tongue thrust				

Contd...

Contd...

S. No.	Test	3 months	6 months	9 months	12 months
	• *Feeding—type:*				
	– Position				
	– Tolerance to feed				
	– Choking spells				
VIII. Voluntary activity					
1.	*Gross motor:*				
	Sit-head erect—3 months				
	Prone—Weight on forearm—3 months				
	Sit-head steady—3 months				
	Prone—Head 90°—4 months				
	Supine-pulled to sit-no lag—4 months				
	Sup/Post Rolls both ways—5 months				
	Sit-Sits erect momentarily—6 months				
	Standing—bears weight 6 months				
	Sit-Sits steadily—7 months				
	Comes to hands and knee—7 months				
	Prone-crawling—8 months				
	Prone-raise and lower from sit—9 months				
	Standing—Cruises—11 months				
	Standing—walks few steps (11–13 months)				
2.	*Fine Motor:*				
	Reflex grasp—0–4 months				
	Palmar grasp—4–8 months				
	Ulnar grasp—4–8 months				
	Control from shoulder—6 months				
	Lateral pinch—8 months				
	Deliberate release—9 months				
	Precise pincer—11 months				
	Opposition—12 months				
3.	*Selfcare:*				
	Finger feeding—9 months				
	Drinks from cup—12 months				
	Grasps spoon—12 months				
	Cooperates in dressing—12 months				

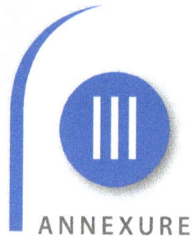

ANNEXURE III

High-risk Follow-up Clinic: Neurological Assessment

Registration No. .... Date: ....
Mother's Name: .... Baby's Name: ....
Date of Birth: .... Corrected age: ....
Ref Dr: ....
Gestation: .... Birth Weight: ....
High-risk factors: ....

3 Months			
Examination	*Status*	*Score normal/ delayed*	*Additional comments*
Supine examination	• Social smile • Antigravity movements • Visual fixation • Visual tracking 180° • Reach • Hand regard • Grasp		
Side lying	Lateral head righting		
Prone	Weight on forearms with head upright		
Pull to sit	Head lag till last 15		
Supported sitting	• Trunk control • Head turning and head control		
Horizontal suspension	Neck and trunk extension		
Protective reaction	Hands forward with prop ups		
Supported standing	Partial weight—bearing intermittent bouts of flexion and extension		
Symmetry			

MUSCLE TONE NORMS

Look for hypotonia/hypertonia, whether symmetric/asymmetric, and record in next table.

Age (month)	Date of Assessment	Age at assessment	Adductor angle	Patient's angle	Popliteal angle	Patient's angle	Dorsi-flexion angle	As assessed	Scarf sign (tick)
0–3 SD			70–94° *84.8 (6.5)		90–100° *100.6 (5.4)		50–59° *55.0 (2.7)		Elbow medial to midline
4–6 SD			90–112° *103.8 (8.0)		100–122° *115.3 (6.1)		52–64° *57.6 (3.3)		Elbow at midline
7–9 SD			101–125° *114.1 (6.2)		110–132° *123.0 (5.6)		55–68° *62.7 (3.4)		Elbow crosses midline (to opposite side)
10–12 SD			118–142° *126.6 (5.3)		120–144° *136.0 (4.0)		58–72° *65.5 (4.6)		Elbow crosses midline

*Indian norms

6 months			
Examination	Status	Score normal/delayed	Additional comments
Supine examination	• Antigravity movements • Reach unilateral • Grasp • Transfer • Foot to mouth		
Side lying	Active rolling		
Prone	• Bears weight on hands, arms extended • Pivots in prone 180° • Reach unilateral • Weight shifting • Dissociation of UL and LL		
Pull to sit	• No head leg • Active neck flexion • UL and abdominal use		
Sitting	• Thoracic extension • Reach unilateral • Active flexion extension • Head control stable		

Contd...

Contd...

Examination	Status	Score normal/delayed	Additional comments
Horizontal suspension	Complete extension		
Protective reaction	• Arms forward • Props on one hand and reach		
Standing	• Sustained weight bearing • Hip behind shoulder, flexed UL extended • Head moves freely		
Symmetry			
9 months			
Supine	Coming to sit		
Prone	• Creeping, crawling • Crawl-sit		
Sitting	• Sitting independently • Protective reactions • Releases small objects • Pincer grasp, pointing		
Standing	Pull to stand, kneels down		
Symmetry			
12 months			
Sitting	• Scribbling—spontaneous/imitates • good transitions • Digital grasp		
Pull to stand	Pull to stand with half knees		
Standing	• Lowering down to sitting • Cruising along furniture • Standing independently • Walking		
Symmetry			

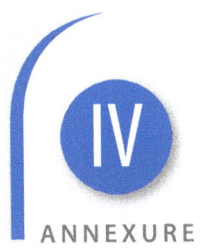

Stimulation Program for Infants

ANNEXURE IV

3–6 MONTHS

- Early stimulation is important for babies at risk for developmental delay- motor development, cognitive functioning, language development, or adaptive functioning.
- All parents want their infants to develop to their maximum potential. Providing the right stimulation at the right time is the key for brain development.
- The greatest single contributor in early stimulation is the mother.
- All babies need stimulation to grow normally, but high-risk babies need planned systematic stimulation to maximize their potential.
- The first year is a very important time for the developing brain. Parents have this golden opportunity to help their baby achieve his or her maximum potential.

Carrying Position
Always carry the child in a comfortable position as shown:

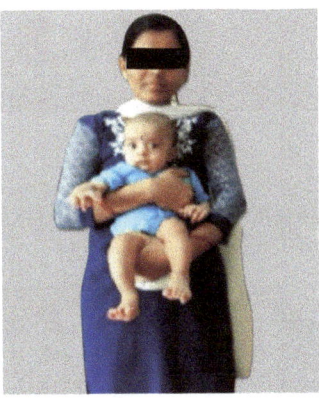

Feeding Position
Always feed your baby in semi-reclining position

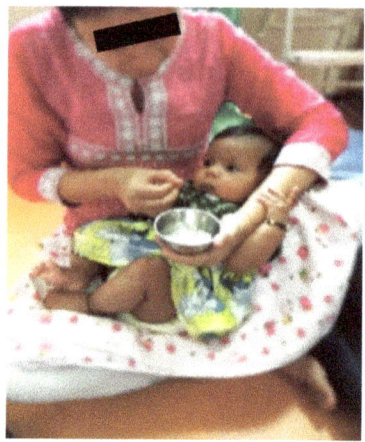

Do not feed in lying down position

To Improve Eye Contact

Hold your baby close to you and talk to the baby looking into his eyes. Always try to maintain eye-to-eye contact, while communicating with your child.

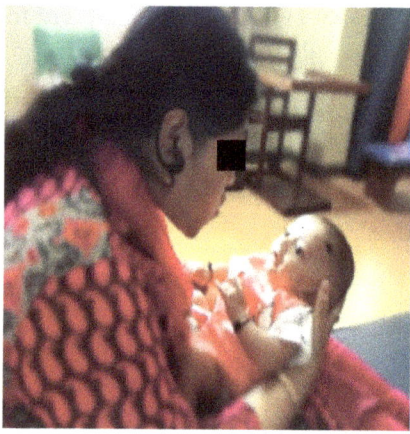

Positioning

Frequently change child's position. Put the child on either side and play with him in side-lying position

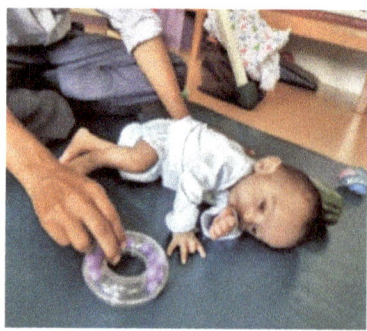

Tummy Time to Improve Neck Control

- Place the child on the stomach, with weight bearing on the elbows.
- Slowly rock the child from side to side.
- Encourage the child to raise the head by showing some attractive toy.
- Move the toy up-down and side to side. Hold your baby close to you to develop sense of bonding.

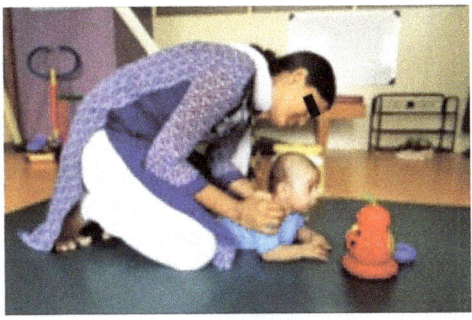

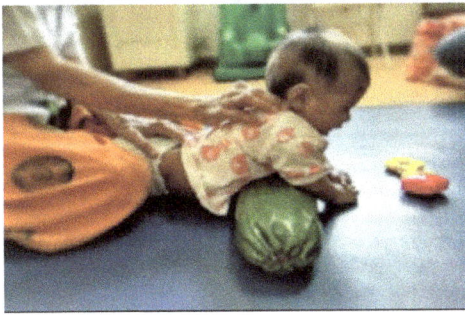

Alternative Tummy Time Positions

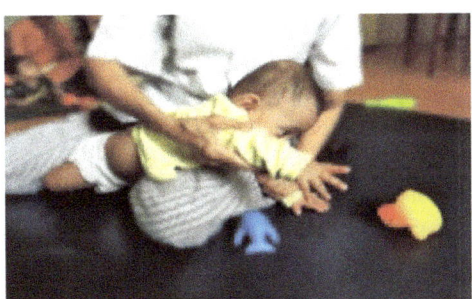

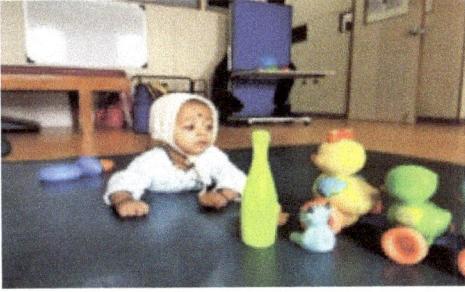

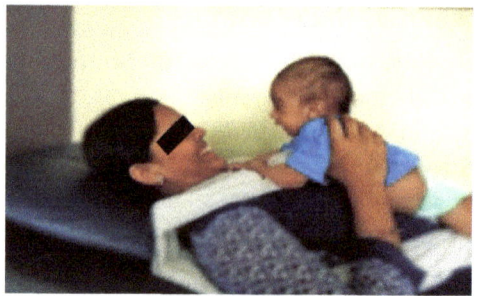

To Encourage Cognitive Development

- Your baby's best toy is you! Interact with the baby as much as possible, while communicating with your baby.
- Allow your baby to experience different sounds, textures, smells and movement.
- Provide safe and hygienic toys for the child, to chew or explore by putting in his mouth.
- Call your child by his name several times.
- Talk to your baby using wide range of vocabulary and lot of expressions.
- Encourage imitation.
- Do actions, sound, and movements which the baby can copy.
- Talk to your baby as you bathe, feed, and dress your baby.
- Let your baby explore. Do not restrict his movements. Allow him to touch and bang the things while playing.
- Use sound producing toys such as bell, rattle or squeaky rubber toys.
- Play games such as peek-a-boo or hide and seek
- Play soft music for your baby. Sing to your baby.

Enjoy your Baby

6–9 MONTHS

- Early stimulation is important for babies at risk for developmental delay- motor development, cognitive functioning, language development, or adaptive functioning.
- All parents want their infants to develop to their maximum potential. Providing the right stimulation at the right time is the key for brain development.
- The greatest single contributor in early stimulation is the mother.
- All babies need stimulation to grow normally, but high-risk babies need planned systematic stimulation to maximize their potential.
- The first year is a very important time for the developing brain. Parents have this golden opportunity to help their baby achieve his or her maximum potential.

Play Activities in Sitting

Make your child sit with one hand support and teach him to take toys with other hand in different directions. This improves his sitting balance.

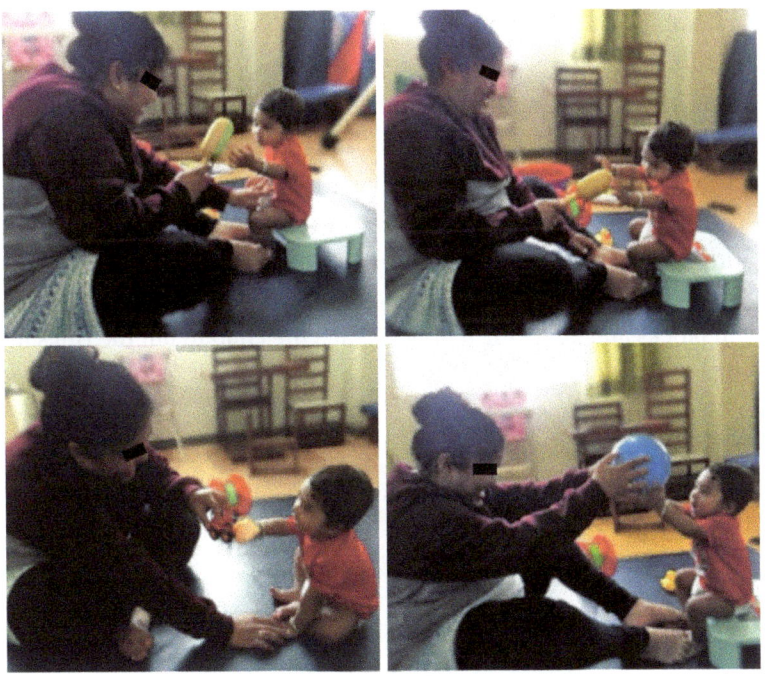

Kneel Standing

Kneel Standing with Stool Support

Make your child stand on his knees with support and play in this position.

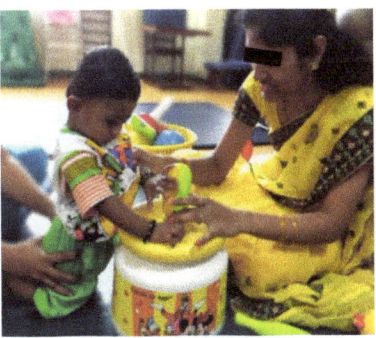

To Encourage Cognitive Development

Cognitive Development in 6-9 Months
- Your baby's best toy is you! Interact with the baby as much as possible.
- Allow your baby to experience different sounds, textures, smells, and movements.

- Provide safe and hygienic toys for the child, to chew or explore by putting in his mouth.
- Call your child by his name several times.
- Talk to your baby using a wide range of vocabulary and lot of expression (Preferably in mother tongue).
- Encourage imitation.
- Do actions, sounds, and movements which the baby can copy.
- Talk to your baby as you bathe, feed, and dress your baby.
- Let your baby explore. Do not restrict his movements.
- Expose the child to different textures. Put your baby on a quilt of different fabrics. The child will be able to see, touch and feel the difference.

Play the games such as filling a container with objects or building a tower with blocks and knocking it down. Teach the child to put the rings in and out of ring stand.

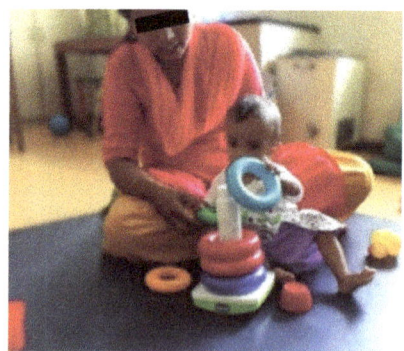

Read to your baby using books with large colorful pictures.

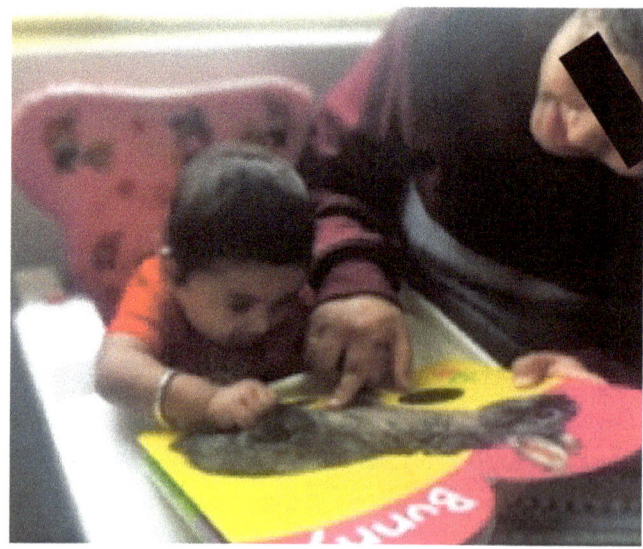

Hide the child's favorite toy under a cloth, while the child is watching. Ask the child to find the toy. Help the child, if he is not able to find it. With this game, the child understands special relationships and problem solving.

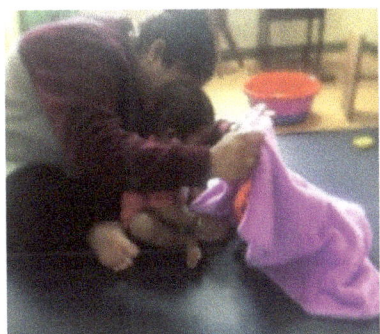
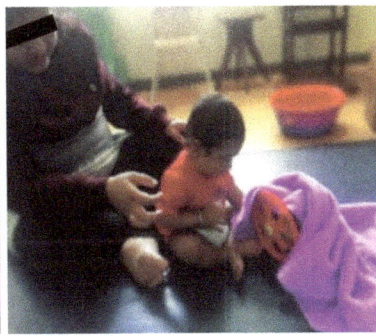

Enjoy Your Baby

Index

Page numbers followed by *b* refer to box, *f* refer figure, *fc* refer to flowchart, and *t* refer to table

A

Adaptive behavior 65
Adductor contracture, amount of 117
Administration procedure 78
Administration time 83
Alternative tummy time positions 179
Amblyopia 50
Amiel-Tison
    method 141, 153
    neurological assessment 57
Ankle
    clonus 169
    dorsiflexion 119*f*
    equines, assessment of 118
    foot orthosis 160
Anthropometry 15
Antivascular endothelial growth factor drugs 48
Arterial tortuosity 44*f*
Ashworth scale, modified 117
Asymmetric tonic neck reflex 166
Ataxia 86
Attention deficit disorders 3
Audiology intervention 143
Auditory brainstem response 25, 27, 28
Auditory cognizance 75
Auditory neuropathy spectrum disorder 22, 30
Auditory steady state response 27, 29
Auditory stimulation 10*f*
Auditory verbal therapist 38
Aural habilitation 37
Automated auditory
    behavioral response 26*t*
    brainstem 24
        response audiometry 26
Axillary suspension 59*f*, 155, 157

B

Baby gymnasium 112*f*
Baby's behavioral repertoire 76
Baby's mental status 72
Baby's mood 72
Baclofen 97
Ballard's gestational age 58
Baroda development screening test 67
Bathing 9
Bayley
    subscales of 81*b*
    test material 82*f*
Behavioral observation 24
    audiometry 27
Bender-Gestalt test 70, 142, 145
Benzyl alcohol 3
Birth asphyxia 138
Birth date, corrected 10
Birth process 22
Birth weight 140*t*
Blood sugar levels 7
Body mass index 151
Bones 115
Borderline intelligence 68
    incidence of 69*f*
Botox injection 161*f*
Botulinum toxin 97, 116, 121, 126
    advantages 123
    disadvantages 123
    dosage of 122, 122*t*
    indication and usage 122
    mechanism of action 122
    method of administration 122
    side effects 123
Brain
    development of 1, 10
    parts of 99
    plasticity of 100
Brainstem evoked response audiometry 10, 11, 28, 29*f*
Breastfeeding 147
Bumbo® chair 107*f*

C

Caloric requirement, increased 54
Catch-up growth 54
Central nervous system 97
Cerebral blood flow 2
Cerebral palsy 56, 86, 96, 115, 116, 139, 140, 160
    children with athetosis 86
    classification of 120
    diagnosis and classification 115

diplegic 96
dyskinetic 96
hemiplegic 96
orthopedic management in 115
quadriplegic 96
severity 87
tone 86
topographic classification of 88*f*, 120
Clostridium botulinum 121
Cochlea, auditory nerve 34
Cochlear implant 35, 36
    parts of 36*f*
Cognition, assessments of 149
Cognitive assessment 147
Cognitive development 101, 181
Cognitive problems 88
Cognitive scale 81
Congenital defects 13
Constipation 89
Cortical blindness 50, 140
Counseling 7
Cranial ultrasonography 7
Crawling 108
    position, small ball in 109*f*
Critical period 99
Crouch gait 124, 125*f*

D

Daily living, activities of 104, 112
Danger signs 90*t*
Dantrolene 97
Deep tendon reflexes 157
Denver developmental screening test 67
Developmental Assessment Scale 15, 67, 72, 73*f*, 139
Developmental quotient 11, 79
Developmental tests 65
Developmental therapy unit 105*f*
Dexamethasone 3
Diazepam 97
Diplegia 87
Disability 135
    diagnosis of 136
Discharge counseling 6
Discharge documentation 7
Discharge planning 6
Discharge screening 7
Disease location 41
Disease stages 41
Distal fashion 101
Draw man test 142

Drooling, control of 113
Dyscalculia 129, 131*f*
Dysgraphia 129, 130*f*
Dyslexia 128, 132*f*
Dyslexic phenotype 132

E

Ear, nose, and throat 16
Early intervention 17, 99
Elbow flexion 126
Electroencephalogram 15
Embryological development 21
Encourage cognitive development 180
Encourage eye-hand coordination 101*f*
Equines 123
Equinovalgus 123
Equinovarus 123
Expressive communication subtest 82
Extensor hypertonia 113*f*
External ear 33
Extraretinal fibrovascular proliferation 41
Eye 154, 155
Eye-hand coordination 100

F

Family
    environmental scale 147, 148
    type of 104
Fetal infant 1
Fine motor subtest 82
Finger flexion 126
Flexed-knee gait 124
Foot problems 123
Fovea sparing partial retinal detachment 43*f*
Fresh, confluent laser marks 48*f*

G

Gait analysis plays 115
Gait pattern classification 120
Gamma-aminobutyric acid 97
Gastroesophageal reflux disease 89
Gastrointestinal tract 97
Genetic problems 100
Gestational age
    appropriate for 131, 142, 146
    small for 14, 129, 131, 142, 146
Gross motor
    function classification system 120
    subtest 83

Growth
    and cognitive development 144
    and development 54
    and nutrition 15
    assessments of 149
    evaluation of 54
    expectations 54
    outcome 54
    patterns 54
    retardation 14
Gymnasium ball 108*f*

H

Hallux valgus 124
Hand
    deformity of 126*f*
    function, development of 111
Head circumference 165
Head control 106, 168
Head growth 60, 154, 155
Hearing aid 34, 34*f*, 35
    parts of 34
    types of 34, 35*f*
Hearing
    assessment 20, 22
        diagnostic tests for 26
    brain 20
    community 37
    detection and intervention 23*t*
    devices 37
    impairment 21, 100, 140
        degree of 20
    neurosensory assessment of 15
    screening protocol 24*fc*
Hearing loss 20, 28, 30, 33
    acquired 22
    causes of 21
    congenital 21
    diagnosis of 33
    fluctuating 30
    hearing aids 35
    mild 30
    risk indicators for 22*t*
    severe-to-profound 33
Hemiplegia 87, 140
    classification of 120
    mild 111
Hemogram 151
Hemorrhage, intraventricular 139
High morbidity 14
High-density lipoprotein 151

High-risk clinic 15*fc*
    functions of 14
    organization of 13
High-risk infant 13, 86
    development in 141
    gestation of 140*t*
High-risk neonates 138
    development of 138
High-risk team 18
Hip
    abduction with knee 118*f*
    dislocation 124
        progressive 117
    displacement 125
    joint 117
    subluxation 124
    surveillance 125
Home-based stimulation program 106
Human figure drawing 70, 142
Hygiene, maintenance of 8
Hyperbilirubinemia 139
Hypertonia 60
    abnormal 59*f*
Hypotonia 60, 63
Hypotonic infant 87*f*

I

Improve eye contact 178
Infant and toddler development, Bayley scales of 81
Infant development, Bayley scales of 74, 84, 139
Infant's developmental assessment 74
Inner ear 34
Inteligence quotient, distribution of 146*t*
Intellectual disability 86
Intelligence quotient 141, 145, 146, 148, 160
    determinants of 148*t*
    maternal education and 56*f*
Intelligence tests 69
Intensive neonatal care 18
Intrinsic growth retardation 54
Ionic calcium 7
Isolation 8

J

Joint 115
    contracture 117
    family 105
Jump knee gait 123

K

Kangaroo mother care 4, 9, 9*f*
Knee
   extension 119*f*
   flexion deformity 124
   joint 117
Kneel standing 181
   with stool support 181
Kneeling position 109
Kuppuswamy scale 139

L

Language 65
   clusters 80
   disorders 86
   scale 81, 82
Laser therapy 49, 52
Laser treatment 47
Lateral propping reaction 169
Lateral propping reflex 61*f*
Learning disabilities 128
   diagnosis of 128
   early diagnosis 133
   high risk of 128
   incidence 128
   prediction 132
   signs for 133
   specific 133
   treatment 134
Learning social skills 129
Legs in spastic infant 87*f*
Lever arm dysfunction 119
Light 2
   pursuit of 166
Lipid profile 151
Low birth newborns 144
Low birth weight 1, 54, 56, 69*f*, 128, 131, 138, 140, 142, 146
   extremely 63, 63*f*, 138
   study 148
   treatment of 49
   typical growth chart of 55*f*
Low cognitive abilities 68
Lower limbs 60

M

Manual dexterity 77, 77*f*
Marked strabismus 166
Massage 8
   oil 8*f*
Mathematics disorder 129
Mathematics score 131*t*
Mean intelligence quotients 142*t*
Medications 3
Memory 76
Meningitis 139
Mental clusters 75*b*
Mental milestones 156, 157
Mental retardation 86, 140, 141
   range of 68
Mental scale 74
Metabolic syndrome 138, 150, 151
   parameters of 151
   predictors of 138
Middle ear 33
   effusion 30
Monoplegia 87, 111
Moro reflex 168
Mortality and morbidity, high postneonatal 14
Motor behavior 65
Motor clusters 75, 75*b*
Motor milestones 65
Motor scale 74, 81, 82
   furniture for 79*f*
Motor skills 104
Movement assessment battery 146
Movement skills 90, 93-95
Muscle 115
   length, assessment of 117
   strength analysis 119
   tone norms 175
Musculoskeletal pathology management 121

N

Neck control 179
Neck extensor
   hypertonicity of 166
   muscles 59*f*
Neonatal care 72
Neonatal intensive care unit 1, 6, 13, 22, 24*fc*, 54, 100, 132, 135, 138, 159
Neonatal reflexes 155, 156, 157
Neonatologist and occupational therapist 170
Nesting 2*f*
Neurobehavior 60
   history for 154, 155, 157
Neurodevelopment 138
   assessment 11, 15, 56
   handicaps 14
   screening test 153
      kit 154*f*

Neurologic diseases 100
Neurologic status 29
Neurological assessment 165, 174
  method of 62
Neuromotor 60
Neurosensory 60, 154
Newborn hearing screening 22
Noise 2
Normalizing tone, techniques for 106
Nutrient deficiencies 89
Nystagmus, sustained 166

O

Occupational therapy 142
  and physiotherapy 104
  intervention 143
Ocular signs, abnormal 57
Ophthalmic examination 52
Ophthalmology intervention 143
Opisthotonos 166
Oral glucose tolerance test 151
Orthopedic surgical intervention 123
Otoacoustic auditory emission 24, 26*t*
Otoacoustic emission 10, 25, 25*f*
Ototoxic medication 21

P

Pain 2
Parachute 169
  reflex 61*f*
Parent-child bonding 104
Parents perspective 159
Pediatric outpatient department 13
Peg board test 77*f*
Pelvic girdle stability 108
Perceptual disorders 86
Persisting plus disease 49*f*
Personal social behavior 65
Phenylephrine 45
Phenylketonuria 20
Physical therapy 101
Planning discharge 6
Plus disease 44
Polycystic ovarian syndrome 151
Pooja bell 10, 15
  response to 166
Poor dental hygiene 89
Popliteal angle 59*f*
Portage Early Education Program 68
Post-botulinum toxin protocol 122
Preterm baby 2
  health status 9
Preterm infant 89, 136

Psychometric assessment 73
Psychometric properties 78, 83
Pupillary dilatation 45

Q

Quadriplegia 87
Qualitative and quantitative assessment 63

R

Radiation 4
Range of motion, analysis of 117
Ranibizumab 49
Raval's social maturity scale 70
Raven's progressive matrices 149
Reaction, support 168
Reading disorder 128
Receptive communication subtest 82
Recordkeeping 17
Rectus femoris spasticity, assessment of 118
Reflexes 60, 90, 91, 93, 94, 154, 157
Refractive errors 50
Respiratory distress 139
  syndrome 52
Retina, examination of 45
Retinal detachment 44
  partial 41
Retinopathy of prematurity 7, 11, 39, 49, 52
  classification of 40
  epidemic
    first 39
    second 39
    third 39
  epidemiology 39
  incidence of 52, 53*f*
  laser, guidelines for 47
  pathophysiology of 40
  posterior 44
  prevalence of 39
  risk factors for 40
  screening for 44
  stages of 53*t*
  surgical management of 49
  treatment for 46
  zones of 41*f*
Retinopathy, extent of 44
Ridge 42*f*
  posterior to 48*f*
  with popcorn vessels 42*f*
Right hip dislocation 125*f*
Rodda and Graham's classification system 120

S

Scarf sign 58
School performance 146
Scoliosis 125
Seizure 86, 88, 139
  disorder 14, 140
Senses 20, 39
Sensory
  auditory nerve 34
  function 20
  impairment 88
  motor integration 172
Septicemia 52, 139
Serum
  bilirubin 7
  electrolyte 7
  triglycerides 151
Setting-sun sign 166
Shoulder adduction 126
Silfverskiöld test 118, 119f
Silverman's score 139
Skills, development of 82
Social and environmental factors 142
Social play 96
Social skills 91-93, 95, 96
Social worker 16
Sociodemography 147
Soft tissue releases 121
Spastic cerebral palsy 60f
Spastic diplegia 120, 140
Spastic infant toe walking 62f
Spastic quadriplegia 140
Spasticity, reduce 97t
Special child 136
Speech
  and language problems 88
  audiometry 28
  therapy 101
Spontaneous asymmetrical tonic neck reflex 60f
Spontaneous motor activity 167
Standard deviation 142
Stanford-Binet
  intelligence scale 69
  test 141
Stimulation kit 102f
Stimulation program 156, 177
Strabismus 50
Stress disorders 3
Supported walking 110f
Supportive humanized care, developmentally 4

Synaptic connections 99f
Syphilis 21

T

Tactile stimulation 3, 4f
Tardieu scale, modified 116
Tendo-Achilles
  left 124f
  weakness 124
Tendons 115
Therapeutic exercises 104
Therapeutic program 114
Therapy plan 106
Thomas hip flexion test 117
Three-dimensional gait analysis 115
Thumb
  adduction 126
  in-palm deformity 126
Tizanidine 97
Toddler development-bayley 81
Tone 116
  active 58f
  and posture 94, 95
  passive 58f
Tonic neck reflex, asymmetrical 96, 106
Topographic classification 87
TORCH 22
Total cerebral tissue volume 3
Total retinal detachment 43f
Toxoplasmosis 21
Transient evoked otoacoustic emission 25
Transient tone abnormalities 63, 63f
Triplegia 87
Trivandrum development screening test 67
Trunk
  dorsal extension of 168
  ventral flexion of 168
Tummy time 106

U

Umbrella term 86
Unilateral cochlear implant 37f
Upper limb 60, 126

V

Ventilator room 2
Very low birth weight 6, 100
Videographic gait analysis 115

Vision 39
    deficits 86
    neurosensory assessment of 15
    primarily 20
Visual attention 101
Visual cognizance 75, 76*f*
Visual impairment 39, 100
    causes of 50
Visual observational gait analysis 115
Visual problems, therapy for 101
Visual reinforcement audiometry 27
Visual stimulation 9*f*
Visual testing 18

Vitreoretinal surgery 49
Vulnerable child syndrome 136

W

W sitting 64*f*
Walking with posterior walker 110*f*
Wechsler intelligence scale 70, 146
Well baby clinic 13, 24*fc*
Weschler's intelligence scale 145, 147
World Health Organization 20, 56
Wrist flexion 126
Written expression, disorder of 129

EU GSPR Authorised Reprsentative
Logos Europe, 9 rue Nicolas Poussin
1700, La Rochelle, France
Phone: +33 (0) 6 67 93 73 78
E-mail: contact@logoseurope.eu